WILL MY BABY
BE NORMAL?

WILL MY BABY BE NORMAL?

Everything You Need to Know

About Pregnancy

JONATHAN SCHER, M.D.

and CAROL DIX

The Dial Press

NEW YORK

LIBRARY OF CONGRESS CATALOGING IN PUBLICATION DATA

Scher, Jonathan.
  Will my baby be normal?

  Includes index
1. Pregnancy. 2. Childbirth. I. Dix, Carol.
II. Title.
RG525.S383 1983   618'.2   82-22234
ISBN 0-385-27651-6

Published by
The Dial Press
1 Dag Hammarskjold Plaza
New York, New York 10017

Copyright © 1983 Jonathan Scher, M.D.

To my wife, Brenda, and my daughters, Amanda and Robyn.

Contents

Introduction

Most likely you are reading this book because you know, or hope, that you are pregnant. I would like to think that some of you are also reading it before you even try to get pregnant. I believe the majority of women today are approaching their pregnancies in a new and enlightened fashion. This pregnancy is very important to you, and the eventual child will mean a great deal to both you and your husband. Consequently you want to do everything possible to ensure the health and safety of this baby.

Realistically it is much less likely than ever before in history that your pregnancy is accidental; and much more likely that the pregnancy was not only very much wanted but that the baby will be deeply and securely loved. Many women planning or contemplating a pregnancy will have already had several years of working, of career development, travel, or just accumulated life experience behind them, and this first step into a completely different way of life is not going to be taken lightly.

I took many things into consideration in preparing a book on pregnancy for today's woman. I wanted to provide you with the most up-to-date information but also with the sort of information you want to acquire. Most young women in their late twenties or early thirties (not to mention those in their late thirties or early forties) about to embark on their first (or a subsequent) pregnancy, worry that by postponing motherhood until so "late" they will run into some serious problem. Although during the last few years we have witnessed escalating rates in the numbers of "late" first-time mothers, some women still suffer guilt from the feeling that they should have married young and had their children first, just as their mothers and grandmothers did. The figures on the decline in fertility and the increase in the occurrence of Down's syndrome (Mongolism), in "late" mothers appear often in the press, and an obstetrician often hears them quoted back to him or her by anxious young women who are newly pregnant.

I have, therefore, subtitled this prenatal-care book for today's woman "Everything You Need to Know About Pregnancy," and I have titled it with that secret, often stifled, always deeply felt question in the mind of any woman who is, or will be, pregnant: "Will My Baby Be Normal?" After "What sex Is it?" this must be the most common question asked. Until very recently all pregnant parents had to wait the full 9 months, or till birth, to find out whether their baby was healthy and normal. The title of the book, I hasten to add, is not meant to instill in you any fear or foreboding. Rather the opposite. It is to indicate my awareness of your concerns and anxieties, plus the fact that I will be addressing myself to the most pertinent questions in your pregnancy.

You should find the book reassuring. Its attitude is positive and its message exhilarating. Today there are very few problems of pregnancy and birth that cannot be dealt with, prevented, remedied, or cured by the most up-to-date techniques in obstetrical medicine.

As an obstetrician, gynecologist, researcher, and teacher who has worked in hospitals over the world and who is now settled both in a joint Manhattan private practice and on the staff of the renowned Mount Sinai Hospital in New York, it has taken me several years to develop the idea of a completely up-to-date and comprehensive prenatal-care book that would be written from your angle rather than mine. Time and again, mature, worldly wise, highly educated women have asked me to recommend a book about pregnancy that would not compromise their intelligence or try to fudge issues with platitudes. They wanted to be abreast of obstetric work that I was performing or might have to do. They wanted to understand terminology and techniques if they heard something new.

Not to denigrate my competition in the book world, but I saw that there was no such book. Then in the spring of 1981 I met writer Carol Dix, a woman in her mid-thirties who had written for many years on medical and social subjects for women, and who had recently had two babies. Our ideas and attitudes seemed to meld and so this book was produced. It has been a labor of love and hard work squeezed in, for me, among my normal obstetric duties, teaching in the hospital, night deliveries, emergency caesarean sections and, for Carol, among the time limits imposed by her young children.

Neither of us is a heavily political animal, but we seem to share an innate sense of feminism and of the respect with which women deserve to be treated. Our agent, Jane Gelfman, and our editor, Joyce Johnson, have shared with us the enthusiasm and downright excitement about this book. Whoever would have thought that new developments in obstetrics would be so fascinating? Everyone involved with me on this book seems to agree that the unfolding story of obstetric care today is breathtaking, uplifting, and differs widely from the traditional approach.

I am not advocating one particular method over another (other than the best). Nor am I beating any drum against possible mistreatment or mismanagement of women in hospitals or by their doctors. I am a physician and obviously write from the point of view of my own skill and experience. If I believed that all women could give birth in the most satisfactory manner, for both mother and baby, at home, helped by husband and paramedics, I would say so. But the perspective of this book is away from the often needlessly negative attitude that the medical world is out to "spoil" a woman's natural and harmonious birth process, or that doctors are notoriously only occupied in obstetrics for motives of greed or power over women.

You should discover in this book the incredible, far-reaching work and new developments that are being tried out and, in some cases, practiced by doctors whose aim is for your happiness and pleasure during pregnancy and birth; but, more so, whose real goal is to produce 100 percent healthy, happy, and wonderfully normal little babies, to eliminate the tragic births of either mentally or physically handicapped children who can bring such anguish or impose such burdens on parents and immediate families, when really we now have the knowledge and equipment to eradicate most of such "mistakes" that nature can produce.

These days the majority of us are having smaller and smaller families. If you come to parenting at a reasonably advanced age, the likelihood is that you will have one, maybe two, children. And you want to be guaranteed, if possible, that your one or two babies will have every chance to be healthy and normal.

In bygone years people procreated as nature, love, or duty dictated. Women produced many children, but they also had many miscarriages. Of the babies born alive, many would not survive the first year of life; some were born with health problems and others with mental disorders. In those days women gave birth to quantity in the hope of having one or two children of quality. Today, all we are concerned about is the quality.

Conceptions are at best a random draw and, as you can read in the section on genetics at the end of Chapter 1, we all carry some faulty genetic material around with us. If a faulty gene is matched with a similar one in your partner, then the offspring can bear the evidence. But even if your randomly drawn conception comes up with healthy genes, we no longer live in an ideal world where the air is pure, the food fresh and uncontaminated. So you must approach the months of pregnancy with special care, as you will read about in Chapters 1 and 2.

There are other factors to be considered in a late-twentieth-century pregnancy. You must be aware of what problems drugs, social or medical, can cause in a pregnancy; and of the effects of the common social addictions, cigarettes, alcohol, and popular soft drugs such as marijuana. Many women will come to this pregnancy after a fairly long history of different contraceptive methods, maybe previous pregnancies that either miscarried or were aborted when a decision was made that this was not the right time to have a child. And you will want to know the effects, if any, this past history will have on your chances for a normal, healthy pregnancy. You will find the answers to these questions and more in Chapter 1.

Finally, a note of further explanation about my particular emphasis—that we can almost guarantee healthy normal babies today—and why I set great store and faith in the skill and experience of our modern obstetricians, particularly those working in the major teaching hospitals in our cities. The hospitals may not be the most beautiful, but the work carried out there is inspiring and should give you utmost confidence.

In the last ten years a quiet revolution, of which you are probably unaware, has been going on in the field of obstetrics. The revolution is in the shift of emphasis away from maternal care during pregnancy and labor, to what we call "fetal care." This means that your doctor will approach your pregnancy as though the fetus were his or her patient, and everything possible will be done to ensure that that fetus is healthy, normal, and is faring as well as it should according to length of gestation, weight, your condition, and all the other mitigating factors that you will be reading about in Chapters 3 and 4.

In obstetric circles the last ten years have become known as the "decade of the fetus." This does not mean you will be sacrificed for the health of the baby. But it does mean we now have more access to the fetus, and more actual knowledge of what is happening inside of you during pregnancy and labor than at any other point in history. Consequently, you will not be forced or encouraged to hold on to a baby that is severely damaged or abnormal, unless you specifically wish to.

When you read here of the many terms and techniques that

will concern you, I hope you will understand that they have been developed for the greater benefit of your baby and, therefore, of you and your husband. Maybe you have already heard about ultrasound, the sonographic device that enables us to see a picture of the baby on a TV-like screen at most stages of the pregnancy from as early as 8 weeks. Maybe you have heard of amniocentesis (particularly if you are thirty-five or over), which is the test performed on the amniotic fluid by which we can determine if your baby has any severely debilitating genetic or chromosomal disorder. But you are also going to come across other terms that may sound weird and mysterious, such as: antepartum fetal heart rate monitoring, nonstress testing, contraction stress testing, estriol level testing, genetics counseling, chromosomal testing, alpha-fetoprotein testing, fetoscopy, fetal scalp blood sampling, and so on and on. So much testing! you might exclaim.

Of course, all these tests are not administered in all pregnancies. The majority still pass without drama or incident; you will be weighed and your urine sample will be tested at each doctor visit—just as your own mother was probably treated. But if yours should prove to be a pregnancy with a problem, you will be greatly relieved to know that the medical experience gained, particularly in the last 10 to 15 years, should minimize the danger and potential harmful effect both for your baby and for you.

Maternal complications are fast becoming a problem of the past in pregnancy and labor. Yet once upon a time the average woman was lucky to survive each pregnancy. In the same way, the figures at present for the number of perfectly normal, healthy babies born stands at a 98 percent likelihood of everything being fine. Within the next few years, therefore, we can feel confident, with the speed of new developments and improvements, that even this ratio will be increased to nearly 100 percent. The 1980s are certainly not a bad time to be having, or considering having, a baby. So do let me wish you luck and happiness with this pregnancy.

Dr. Jonathan Scher
Mount Sinai Hospital
New York City

WILL MY BABY

BE NORMAL?

CHAPTER

1

In the Beginning...

You may already know you are pregnant and have your first doctor's appointment booked; you may be wondering whether you are pregnant and have decided it is time to read up on the subject; or you may be hoping that time and nature have been on your side and that a conception has taken place.

Knowing about your pregnancy, understanding what is happening to you, and appreciating what your doctor is talking about or doing will help make the journey toward birth that much more rewarding and fascinating.

The thrill of discovering that you are pregnant may be overshadowed to some degree by the mystery of what will be happening to your body, and the need to feel confident that your baby is in fact all right in the uterus. So, in this first chapter, the kinds of anxieties that particularly perplex women in the 1980s will be explained and the various problems that might be involved will be discussed frankly. This should help you approach your pregnancy with a positive, happy attitude and enable you to discuss your own worries with your obstetrician.

So let me begin at the beginning and look at what kind of

woman is best suited for pregnancy and see if there are any factors that actually contraindicate pregnancy for you.

When are you considered healthy enough to be pregnant?

Basically if you have no communicable diseases and have had a thorough checkup with your doctor to test for anemia, heart disease, or diabetes; if you are clear of influenza or common colds; have had vaginal disorders such as Monilia (thrush) or Trichomonas treated; then there is very little to worry about. You should make sure your system is clear by at least 1 month of all drugs, whether they were for medical or social use. If you are on any maintenance therapy—say for migraine, for an underactive thyroid, or for heart disease—tell your physician you are contemplating pregnancy and you will be advised whether you may adjust or discontinue the drug.

You should be free for at least 2 months from any form of contraceptive (even spermicides) and at least 3 months away from an abortion or spontaneous miscarriage. From now on, you should try to eat well, exercise, stabilize your life style, cut down on heavy drinking and if possible on cigarette smoking, and aim for a healthy, optimistic attitude toward this future exciting event in your life.

If a patient came to me before she tried to get pregnant to ask about her health and whether she was in condition to carry a child, I would run through a chronology of her previous illnesses and current medications. I would ask her to describe to me all the nonprescription drugs she takes daily, or occasionally, such as cold or antacid remedies, and what social drugs she uses. Alcohol, cigarettes, and occasional use of marijuana will be significant to your pregnancy only if they have been used in excess. If they are discontinued before you attempt pregnancy, they will not be a cause for concern. It is very important to be aware of your past medical history, and your current vices, so that both you and your doctor can prevent any problems.

Your previous induced abortions and spontaneous miscarriages are significant whether you are taking the Pill and when you intend to stop, whether you have an IUD in place or have been using spermicides.

If you are a teenager, there may be significant problems to watch for; if you are over thirty-five, your pregnancy will be managed carefully. If you are very short, under five feet tall; if your prepregnant weight is more than 20 percent under or over the average; if you have had over five full-term pregnancies; or if you have a history of prolonged infertility and have been on hormone therapies, your doctor will take these factors into account when determining the management of a future pregnancy.

As for common illnesses and their effect on pregnancy or conception, the main consideration will be the type of medication you are using. A woman came to see me recently who was taking antibiotics and was trying to get pregnant. What should she do? By mentioning the problem to me, she took the first correct step.

You must be careful in the second half of any menstrual cycle in which you could get pregnant not to take social drugs or over-the-counter medications without first consulting your doctor. If the problem is drugs that are being prescribed for your own health, make sure your doctor is aware of your pregnancy and that he or she investigates the dosage and possible alternatives.

I recently managed the pregnancy of a young woman with leukemia. Throughout her pregnancy she was taking the highest doses of cytotoxic drugs (which may have an effect on the fetus). I went completely against the book in one sense; that it was a calculated risk, as the mother's life was in jeopardy. Do you know, the baby was born a few weeks ago and despite that bombardment of medications it was perfect.

5

WILL MY BABY BE NORMAL?

HEIGHT	WEIGHT
4'10"	104
4'11"	107
5'0"	110
5'1"	113
5'2"	116
5'3"	118
5'4"	123
5'5"	128
5'6"	132
5'7"	136
5'8"	140
5'9"	144
5'10"	148
5'11"	152
6'0"	156

The table shows the standard weight for height of medium build women 25 years and older. (Younger women should deduct one pound per year of age). The table has been adjusted to your normal height wearing low-heeled shoes. Your doctor can tell from this standard whether you are very much under or over-weight when pregnancy begins.
Chart courtesy of Metropolitan Life Insurance Company.

You do not want to become inadvertently pregnant while still taking such drugs as: the Pill (the hormones can cause masculinization of a female baby's genitals and problems with bony development); antibiotics such as streptomycin or tetracycline (never use up any leftover antibiotics in the medicine cabinet to try to clear a sore throat); antithyroid drugs; diuretics; high-dose vitamins; sleeping tablets with barbiturates; diet pills with amphetamines; or tranquilizers. If you should find yourself

6

pregnant, stop using the medication immediately and inform your doctor exactly what you have been taking and for how long, but do not panic. It is only recently that we have been able to diagnose pregnancy as early as 6 days before the first missed period and, prior to such times, women were frequently discovered treating symptoms of nausea, tiredness, and a general feeling of being unwell as influenza rather than pregnancy. Many women took antibiotics then for several weeks into a pregnancy and have had perfectly normal, healthy babies. But if you are reading this chapter in an attempt to be best prepared for a future pregnancy, you will know the cautious steps to take in the second half of any menstrual cycle in which you may become pregnant.

What about your husband's or prospective partner's health?

Sometimes women or their husbands ask me if the man's state of health has any effect on the pregnancy or fetus. In general, the answer is no, unless he is over fifty-five, in which case he should be tested for possible chromosomal problems, as he may contribute to a baby born with Down's syndrome (see page 78). Pregnancy should be avoided for varying periods of time (depending on the physician's advice) if the potential father has been given any radioactive treatment, e.g. radioactive iodine for thyroid disease, or a cytotoxic drug used in cancer treatment. We know little as yet about the effect of drugs, medical or social, on sperm, though it is known that chronic use of cigarettes or marijuana may affect a man's sperm count and make conception more difficult. I would advise for safety's sake that your husband be off all drugs and, if he is taking any prescription medication, that you ask his doctor and yours about the possibility of its affecting the fetus.

When should you begin to consider your health and condition for pregnancy?

We tend to believe that conception happens magically one night, sedately in the bedroom, erotically in the woods, or drunkenly after a party. But, as we still do not know exactly when the egg and sperm actually meet and unite after intercourse, this union is just as likely to be taking place as you step onto the subway, sit in the Laundromat, or drink your coffee at the office.

A woman used to become suspicious only maybe 3 weeks after the event, by which time her period would be rather late. Within 4 weeks of ovulation, she might begin to feel nauseated, notice that her breasts were swollen, or feel a tingling sensation in the nipples. She would go for a pregnancy test, maybe 4 to 6 weeks after ovulation and conception. At that point, with a doctor's confirmation in her hand, she would begin to be concerned about the growing life inside her and how she should modify her own life style for the baby's safety.

However, her pregnancy had in fact already existed for 4 to 6 very important weeks. The first 56 days (8 weeks) of embryonic life—that is, counting from ovulation and fertilization—are one of the most vital periods of fetal development. Called the period of organogenesis, it is when the fundamental formation of the organs takes place. (Doctors usually count a pregnancy from the first day of your last period because no one knows, as I have just explained, when conception actually takes place. But that form of dating adds 2 weeks to an embryo's life. You will generally hear it said, therefore, that the first 12 weeks, the whole of the first trimester, is the overall danger period.)

One of the greatest advances in prenatal care has been the discovery of an efficient very early pregnancy test. This new blood test, which measures the level of HCG (human chorionic gonadotrophin), the hormone that indicates pregnancy, can now give a positive result 8 days after ovulation, that is, 6 days before you would expect to miss a period. I am not saying that every woman will get a pregnancy test so early. Many will still not suspect they are pregnant until they have missed a period and begin to feel some of the sensations I have described; and some will not miss periods for a few months. But when you appreciate the significance of fetal growth and development in those days and weeks immediately after conception, you will see why an early confirmation is advisable. You will want to avoid using any drugs or medications that might harm the minuscule embryo.

Let me explain what is happening inside you once the released egg has been fertilized by a sperm, has successfully traveled down the Fallopian tube, and has become implanted in the uterine wall (all of which takes 6 to 7 days after ovulation). The implanted egg is kept alive at first by the corpus luteum, which is a cystic structure that remains in the ovary after ovulation. It ensures the hormones necessary for the pregnancy to survive and cause changes needed for the embryo's growth and nourishment, until the placenta takes over—sometime between the eighth and fourteenth week after fertilization. The exact moment when anything that is absorbed into your bloodstream may be absorbed into the embryo's bloodstream is uncertain. And although we are not completely sure about which substances cross the placenta, or when the embryo begins to depend on the placenta for its life support, we do know that the embryo is vulnerable from the moment of fertilization on.

The fertilized egg develops incredibly rapidly in the first 4 weeks, taking shape less like a human baby at this stage than like some amphibious sea creature. It is a crescent-shaped structure with marks where eyes, ears, arms, and legs will one day develop and grow. If you want to see pictures of the earliest embryonic stages (and the full fetal development as well), I recommend that you take a look at a remarkable book called *A Child Is Born*, by Lennart Nilsson (Delacorte Press, 1977). Nilsson is a Swedish photographer who gives a wonderful portrait of this early stage of development, and will convince you, if my words fail to, why you should be careful of what you put into your body.

For example, at the end of the third week (after ovulation) the nervous system starts to develop. There is a long tunnel, or tube (the neural tube), which later will develop into the brain, spinal cord, and nerves. The embryo also has a primitive mouth, face, and throat. There is gill-like tissue forming the beginnings of the lower jaw and throat.

On the eighteenth day, the eyes and ears start to form.

On the twenty-fifth day, the primitive heart starts beating, very rapidly, 65 times a minute.

On the twenty-sixth day, the limb buds are visible; within a few days, soft paws with a suggestion of fingers can be seen.

On the thirty-first day, the arm buds become hands, arms, and shoulders.

On the thirty-third day, the finger outlines are visible.

On the thirty-seventh day, the tip of the nose is visible, and the eyelids begin to form.

By the sixth week the embryo already has a heart and liver. And, at 8 weeks (still counting from ovulation rather than from the onset of your last period), the embryo becomes a fetus; the corpus luteum has stopped growing and shriveled up; and the fetus begins to depend totally on the placenta for food, oxygen, and cleansing.

By the end of this second month, the buds of twenty baby teeth are in the upper and lower jaws, and the lips and tongue will be formed. The fetus has grown to about an inch long, and its head is bent on the chest. (The head is about one third of the total length of the fetus at this stage.) The brain has just begun to develop.

These first 8 weeks (56 days) are perhaps the most important time in the whole development of the fetus, as all of the structures that will be present when the baby is born 7 months later will have been formed in their primitive stages. The period of "organogenesis" is usually taken to mean the first 12 weeks of pregnancy. From the third month on, the fetus begins to grow, to learn some more human activities, such as tumbling in the amniotic fluid, kicking, even sucking its thumb and hiccuping.

Without being a sensationalist, let me just remind you that the drug Thalidomide—a sedative taken by pregnant women some 30 years ago, which caused limb deformities in their children—was generally taken in the first 39 to 56 days of pregnancy, when women were feeling nauseated or needed help with sleep. So do check with your doctor before taking any social, over-the-counter, or prescribed drug during this period.

What in your past life might affect a future pregnancy?

If you are an older first-time mother you very likely have experimented with various contraceptive methods; you may or may not have had one or more abortions, or one or more spontaneous miscarriages. On top of that, many of us of all ages eat badly, consume too many caffeine-containing drinks, use excess alcohol, smoke heavily, and experiment with soft or hard drugs as escape or entertainment.

Now most of these behavior patterns will have to stop. Whatever you did before this pregnancy, secure in the knowledge that you were only hurting yourself, will have to be approached from a different viewpoint. Even if you are not to "eat for two," certainly whatever you take into your body can and will affect your baby in some way for the next 9 to 10 months. (I date everything to do with the pregnancy from the middle of the cycle when ovulation and conception took place.)

Most of the information I have to give you, however, is reassuring rather than alarming. I do know that such issues are of general concern, so I have tried to be absolutely frank about them. As some women find it hard to ask their doctor personally for this kind of information, I hope I have provided a valuable service.

YOUR PAST AND PERSONAL EXPERIENCES

Contraception

May you conceive immediately on stopping contraception?

Many women now thinking about trying to get pregnant have been using one or more forms of contraception for several years, and are genuinely concerned about the effects various contraceptive methods will have on future childbearing. I am often asked about this. And I do understand that there is a high level of anxiety about the potential harmful effects of the various contraceptive methods—which is not altogether helped by regular sensational stories throughout the media about such-and-such a device causing abnormalities or birth defects.

To put the question into perspective, I would say that if you have any anxiety or nervousness about conception, discuss it with your gynecologist, who will no doubt advise you to wait a full month after stopping the use of any form of contraception. If you find your periods do not return immediately after stopping a particular form of contraception—notably the Pill, intrauterine device, or the progesterone-releasing intrauterine device—then wait a few months until your system returns to normal before really thinking about trying to get pregnant. If you believe your lack of periods is a serious problem, seek your doctor's help *before* you begin to fear you will never conceive.

If your contraceptive device was an IUD—whether a Copper 7, Lippes Loop, Saf-T-Coil, or the progesterone-releasing T-coil—you may in fact try to conceive immediately on its removal, as the IUD only works to prevent pregnancy while it is inserted and has no long-term effects. Once removed, its prior use will not be harmful to a future pregnancy.

If you have been using condoms to prevent pregnancy, there is no inherent danger, and you may try to conceive whenever you so decide. However, if you have been using spermicides alone (creams, jellies, or suppositories) or in conjunction with a mechanical contraceptive device inserted in your vagina (diaphragm or cervical cap), you may be concerned by recent reports that women who conceive while still using spermicides may run the risk of bearing babies with birth defects.

This warning about spermicides is extremely new and contradicts a major study by the Boston University Hospital Drug Epidemiology Unit some 3 years ago, which concluded that there is no evidence to show that women who conceive while still using spermicides show any difference in the number of genetic birth defects, chromosomal defects, malformations, or spontaneous miscarriages, than those women who stopped using them *before* trying to conceive.

However, because the issue is not yet entirely resolved, it would be wise to take the precaution of waiting a full month after using spermicides before attempting a pregnancy. In the interim, use condoms or rely on the rhythm method or practice abstinence. My own feeling is that spermicides have been used for generations and, as so many pregnancies happen not entirely by choice but by the malfunction or misuse of such forms of contraception, any serious association between spermicides and birth defects would have been noticed long ago.

The contraceptive Pill also appears to have *no* long-term harmful effect on a future pregnancy. If you are planning to conceive, I advise you to wait a full month after having stopped taking the Pill, by which I mean, let two menstrual periods pass before attempting a pregnancy, so that your ovulatory system will be functioning properly and your body will be free of synthetic hormones. To prevent a pregnancy during this time, use condoms, or practice the rhythm method. Even though the Pill contains synthetic estrogen and progestogen (the synthetic form of progesterone), there is no evidence that previous consumption of these hormones has any harmful effect on subsequent pregnancies. Large studies have in fact shown no difference in the rate of miscarriages, or of congenital deformities in the offspring of those who had taken the Pill and those who had used other contraceptive devices, or none at all.

What if you become pregnant while taking the Pill?

Fortunately, accidental pregnancies while a woman is taking the Pill continuously and properly are so few as to be almost negligible. But I must caution you to be careful that you use the Pill correctly, especially if you plan to have a baby in the near future.

Should you become pregnant and find that inadvertently you have continued taking the Pill, there is evidence to show that this can lead to congenital abnormalities in your baby (the FDA cites pregnancy as one of the five contraindications for the Pill). So do inform your doctor immediately if this happens to you. In such a situation—since the resulting birth defects can be widespread—you may consider, with your doctor's advice, a therapeutic abortion. If you have taken the Pill while pregnant, there is also the possibility of masculinization of the sex organs of a female fetus.

If you have been taking the Pill for a long time, can it affect your future childbearing?

There is evidence that your fertility *may* be delayed for a few months after you stop taking the Pill—up to 20 percent of Pill takers are affected. Unfortunately it is not always possible to avoid this. If, after stopping the Pill, you do not have menstrual periods in a reasonable length of time (say 6 months), then discuss it with your doctor. He or she will be able to reassure you that all is well; your periods will return of their own accord. Your doctor can induce a period (actually a withdrawal bleed) with a progestogen; or, if you are anxious to conceive, ovulation can be induced with a fertility agent such as Clomid or by using other methods.

Any teenager or woman with a history of missed periods, or amenorrhea (no periods), should not use the Pill, as her reproductive system may be suppressed. Unfortunately it was fashionable some years back to prescribe the Pill to young women with menstrual problems as a panacea. The Pill certainly did not cure their menstrual problems; it merely covered them up.

What happens if you conceive with an IUD in place?

No one knows precisely how IUDs actually work, but they *do* work, though there is a failure rate of 4 to 6 out of every 100 users.

From early animal experiments it was discovered that even a thread of cotton in the uterus would act as a contraceptive. The contraceptive ability of a foreign body in the uterus, therefore, does not depend entirely on what it is or how big it is, just that it is there. Why is an IUD effective? Most likely because the IUD makes the Fallopian tubes, which conduct the egg from the ovary to the uterus, *beat* more rapidly, speeding up the egg's passage down the tubes. A fertilized egg should remain in the tubes at least 6 to 7 days, while preparing to implant in the endometrium. If its journey down the tubes in shortened, the egg hits the endometrium in an immature condition and naturally aborts.

The physical presence of the IUD also apparently reduces the area in the uterus available for implantation of the egg, and attracts certain body cells into the endometrium that may digest the egg.

Why does a pregnancy happen with an IUD in place?

As I mentioned above, the incidence of IUD failure is quite high when compared to that of the Pill. But do not worry. If you conceive with an IUD inserted, you can have it removed if the thread is visible and have a perfectly normal pregnancy.

Or if the thread is not accessible, you can even go to term with the IUD still in place and have a normal birth if you so desire. (Sometimes, removal of the device is impossible if the thread seems to be missing, or if the device is too high up in the uterus.) Your doctor will be able to locate the IUD by testing you with an ultrasound scan. There is always the chance the IUD has been ejected by your body without your realizing it. If you decide to continue the pregnancy with an IUD *in situ*, discuss it carefully with your doctor, as there is an increased risk of miscarriage (a 25 percent chance) and also greater risk of uterine infection. Fortunately, however, congenital damage to the baby is not a problem.

Indeed, I have delivered many babies with the IUD still in the uterus. The fetus is inside a protective balloon (the amniotic sac) before delivery, and the intrauterine device is stuck on the outside of the sac like a piece of gum. The IUD does not come into contact with the fetus, as it is excluded by the developing sac and compressed between the membranes and the uterine wall.

Unfortunately a proportion of IUD pregnancies are ectopic (tubal) pregnancies. Why they happen, we do not know, though the cause may be linked to a failure in the mechanisms I have just described. Possibly a subtle pelvic infection induced by the IUD's presence prior to conception had affected the tubes and caused the ovum to lodge in the infected tube. A tubal pregnancy is abnormal, can never go to term, and usually requires surgery for removal.

Your doctor can diagnose a tubal pregnancy with ultrasound, and with the very sensitive pregnancy tests now available. You may not know you have such a pregnancy, as in 50 percent of these cases a woman has not missed a period by the time she comes to her doctor with symptoms such as low abdominal pain, dizziness, and possibly scanty menstrual bleeding. If you ever have such symptoms see your doctor immediately and be sure to explain that you have an IUD.

In the Beginning . . .

Induced Abortion

Does a history of more than one induced abortion mean you will have greater difficulty conceiving or bearing a child?

There has been much controversy over whether an induced abortion—one you have chosen to bring on rather than one that occurs naturally (which we call "spontaneous abortion," or miscarriage)—increases the rate of future infertility or miscarriage.

Despite the fact that abortion is a legal process and that a large majority of the population regards it as an unfortunate but necessary medical procedure, there is much underlying guilt in many women who have had abortions (especially if they have had more than one) and the fear that somehow their "wrongdoing" will be punished later on when they are *trying* to conceive. I would like to put the issue in perspective so you will not be unduly troubled by such guilt or anxiety. Past abortion and future childbearing really bear very little relation to each other.

One patient of mine, who was newly married and at the airport about to leave with her husband on their honeymoon, telephoned me in state of panic. She was pregnant and did not feel that this soon in the marriage was the right time to begin a family. If she decided to terminate the pregnancy, she asked in desperation, would it affect her future childbearing? They really did want to have children one day. Would an abortion make her infertile, or lead to miscarriages?

Over the last few years, the issue of abortion has become so confused with politics and feminist argument that you may not be aware of the fact that while these arguments rage in the public forum, we in the medical profession have been quietly improving the methods by which abortions are performed, so that now they are not only safe, sure, and legal, but are also unlikely to affect any future pregnancies.

17

The abortion debate in our country may also have clouded some of the basic facts. For example, our own practice is far removed from that of many other nations. In Eastern Europe, abortion has been used as a method of contraception for several years, and many women in those countries have had ten or twelve abortions, without any harmful effects on future *wanted* pregnancies.

The likelihood of a past abortion affecting subsequent wanted pregnancies in the U.S. today is *nil*, as long as the abortion was performed properly by a qualified doctor under clinic or hospital conditions, and at a reasonably early stage in the pregnancy. Having said that, I must add it does hold true that abortions beyond the first 8 weeks of pregnancy, especially a number of such abortions, may increase the risk of future miscarriages, either because of pelvic infection or from stretching of the cervix. In the latter case, the cervix will dilate early in the pregnancy (known as cervical incompetence), which may cause a second-trimester miscarriage. Even that is very unlikely unless you had an extremely traumatic (physical, not psychological) abortion, in which the cervix was forced or torn.

Now, as you will see from the following information about the newer techniques, even these possibilities are being minimized. You run very little risk of any subsequent complications, I would say, if your abortions were performed after the mid-1970s, by which time most doctors in this country had stopped using forcible dilation of the cervix to conduct the operation.

Abortion has become much less hazardous. The complete liberalization of the abortion laws has meant that most women now seek abortions early. They do not wait around in panic or waste precious weeks trying to find someone who will perform an abortion illegally.

For the sake of all women, I do believe in the legalization of abortion. We in the medical profession know only too well from

past experience the sad and often tragic consequences of illegal abortion.

The other reason for improvement in abortion techniques is the availability of the more sensitive pregnancy testing which is done on the blood rather than on the urine and which can diagnose a pregnancy very early (see page 8 on early pregnancy tests). Such early diagnosis has meant that most abortions can now be performed without mechanical dilation of the cervix. Early abortions have become known as "lunchtime abortions." A patient attends an out-patient clinic and is given a local anesthetic in the cervix. After about 10 minutes a fine soft catheter is introduced into the uterus and its contents are aspirated. There is no recognizable fetus up to 9 or 10 weeks of pregnancy, which is easier both on the woman's mind and on the medical staff performing the abortion.

If you are over 10 weeks but under 18 weeks pregnant, we can still avoid much of the stretching of the cervix, by softening it with laminaria (which is, in fact, dried seaweed), put into the cervix overnight. By next morning, your cervix will be open. Or, similarly, we can soften the cervix by placing a prostaglandin suppository up against the neck of the uterus just a few hours before the abortion. With either of these methods we are still able to do a vacuum aspiration abortion without forcible mechanical dilation of the cervix and consequent possible damage. A general anesthetic, however, will be needed.

From 18 to 24 weeks of pregnancy, an abortion is done by intra-amniotic injection. A drug containing urea, prostaglandin, and sometimes saline, is injected directly into the amniotic fluid. For that you would be hospitalized, given the injection, and then you would wait until you started a mini-labor, as the cervix takes several hours to dilate. The process may be slow and more uncomfortable, but you will have what amounts to a normal delivery, and such an abortion will not affect your future childbearing any more than will normal labor.

Abortion techniques may improve even further with the extensive research now being done on the use of prostaglandins. We conducted a research experiment here at Mount Sinai Hospital on prostaglandin abortions. The chemical was given as a vaginal suppository which, after an internal examination of the uterus, was pushed high up in the vagina. The women in the study lay on beds for an hour and were then allowed to walk around. Prostaglandin, a hormone found in the female and male reproductive system, comes into action during the onset of your menstrual period and is responsible for cramps. In just the same way as it works naturally, the prostaglandin suppository is absorbed into the system and produces cramps 15 minutes to 2 hours later, followed by vaginal bleeding within the next 5 hours. None of the women in the study was more than 7 weeks pregnant, and all but one successfully aborted. We hold great hopes for this as a future method of abortion, as it could be done in your *own home*, without any of the inconvenience or embarrassment associated with even out-patient abortions.

How long after a miscarriage or induced abortion should you wait before trying for another pregnancy?

After a miscarriage you should wait at least 3 months before conceiving as there is evidence to suggest that the risk of neural tube defects in the fetus increases if conception takes place within this interval. Beyond that there are no medical reasons why you should not try for another baby after a miscarriage.

If you have recently had an induced abortion, however, the answer to the question really depends on your state of mind. If the abortion was sought for deep personal reasons, however strong your desire may be to have a baby, do give it time— even up to a year afterward—before you try again. You really do not want to have a succession of abortions during a period of personal crisis, as it will only help compound your problems.

Give your body a chance to settle down, and it will slowly help your mind come around to the same point.

Do not panic. Although women begin to fear the end of their fertility around the age of thirty, you still have at least 10 more healthy years in which you can have children without any problems, and within which time you will no doubt find yourself in a situation better suited to parenthood. If you have had a termination because of contraceptive misuse, or because of a state of confusion over the man involved or your own decision to become a parent, do yourself a favor and wait several months before you become pregnant again.

Do tell your doctor, however ashamed or guilty you feel about your history of induced abortions, exactly how many there have been and by what methods they were performed. Although the risk is minimal to subsequent pregnancies, he or she must know for the future care of your health. Your doctor will respect your confidence, and will in no way judge you detrimentally because of this history.

A final word of reassurance to those women who had D & C abortions before the mid-1970s—as I realize I spoke rather freely about the possible danger of dilation of the cervix in the second trimester: There is still much that can be done if the mouth of the cervix should open up early in a pregnancy.

First, your doctor may suspect and be on the lookout for such an occurrence because of your past history; especially if it has happened to you in a previous pregnancy, or if you had a late abortion. Second, cramps or bleeding in the middle trimester (after 12 weeks) may be a sign of the cervix opening. Third, if on repeated vaginal examinations the doctor notices that the cervix is shortening or dilating, then he or she will take some preventive measures. Ultrasound examination can help confirm the clinical evaluation.

You may find your strenuous activities, such as exercise or travel, curtailed, and it may be suggested you give up working for a few months. Your doctor might suggest extra bed rest, which is important as a precaution against miscarrying. Full sexual intercourse (penetration) should be stopped, although other sexual activity, including orgasm, is permitted.

If you are getting cramps which could open the cervix even further, you may be given some new preventive agents, called beta-mimetics, which are used to stop premature labor (see page 221). These can be used after the twentieth week of pregnancy, will settle the cramps or bleeding, and will not harm the baby.

Once the bleeding or cramping has been controlled, it may then be decided to strengthen and close up the cervical opening (mouth of the uterus) with a cervical cerclage procedure commonly known as the Shirodkar stitch. The stitch can be placed at any time during the pregnancy, but it is usually done between the twelfth and twenty-eighth week (see page 160).

Miscarriages

Why do spontaneous miscarriages happen?

If you have had one or more spontaneous abortions (the terms *miscarriage* and *abortion* are synonymous, though popularly *abortion* implies an induced end to pregnancy), it may be heartening to know that out of the 5 to 10 million conceptions a year in America, at least one third or between 2 to 3 million end up in spontaneous abortion. So you are most certainly not alone. No one can ever know the exact figure, for many abort soon after conception, even before the mother suspects she is pregnant—or a miscarriage may just seem like a heavy period.

Another 1 million conceptions are terminated, and that leaves us with the figure of about 3 million live births per year in this country.

If you have recently suffered a spontaneous miscarriage, you no doubt are concerned about what it means. Will you miscarry again? Will you ever be able to give birth to a healthy, normal baby? Well, as many as 15 to 20 percent of normal women miscarry in their first pregnancy and, of these early abortions, up to 40 percent have been shown to be due to chromosomal abnormalities. This is not meant to alarm you, nor to imply that future pregnancies will be subject to similar chromosomal defects. Chromosomal abnormalities can come about because of genetic predisposition in you or your husband; or because of some environmental factor that has affected the fertilization of this particular ovum.

So a first miscarriage is nothing to be too alarmed about. You will most likely go on to have a perfectly healthy normal pregnancy, though it may seem unattainable at the time. There is no need for any special tests or investigations, but when you visit your obstetrician on the next pregnancy, make sure he or she knows of the previous miscarriage. Only when you have had two recurrent spontaneous miscarriages—one after the other in successive pregnancies—will your doctor want to begin special investigations. There are several tests that can be done at that time to help your physician advise and guide your future attempts at childbearing.

What can be done about repeated miscarriages?

If you fall into the group of recurrent spontaneous aborters (two or more miscarriages in successive pregnancies), it is vital that you consult your doctor or attend one of the special clinics that are being set up for this purpose. Here at Mount Sinai Hospital our clinic is called the Pregnancy Support Clinic. Ask your doctor if such a clinic exists near you and request referral, even if it means quite a long journey. So much more is known now about the causes of spontaneous abortion that you will find any necessary travel well worth the effort.

The first part of the investigation will be to test the possibility of *hormonal* causes. Let me explain. The ovum, once released and fertilized by the sperm, having traveled the length of the Fallopian tube, nests in the uterus and is kept alive for the first 12 to 14 weeks not by the placenta, which has not yet fully developed, but by a yellow yolklike structure called the corpus luteum, which is present in the ovary after ovulation and provides the egg with the necessary hormones and nutrition until the placenta finally takes over.

Before you try for another pregnancy, your physician will want to test the effectiveness of the corpus luteum to see if your hormone levels are adequate in the nonpregnant state. This is done by assessing your menstrual cycle. If the time between your periods is normal, then the hormone levels are probably adequate, despite a history of miscarriages. You will be asked to keep a chart to see if your temperature remains slightly elevated for 14 days after ovulation. On a certain day in your cycle, your obstetrician may also take a sampling of the endometrium (lining of the womb) which a pathologist will be able to assess.

Hormonal levels may also be measured by a blood test from your arm that will show whether the level of progesterone is sufficient for the time of your menstrual cycle. An even newer technique is being developed—using ultrasound pictures of the actual size of the corpus luteum following ovulation.

All the hormone systems in the body are linked, so your doctor will also check for disturbances in any other part of the hormonal network that, theoretically, could help trigger a miscarriage. He or she will look for diabetes (particularly uncontrolled or latent diabetes), or for a thyroid problem. An underactive thyroid, for example, only has a minimal role in disturbing hormonal balance, yet it can be enough to trigger a miscarriage. Thyroid medication is not harmful to a pregnancy, so if the condition were confirmed, it could be treated.

Infections are the next source of a cause for spontaneous abortions. Only recently have infections been identified as playing a major part in recurrent spontaneous abortions. But now that we have this new information at hand, it does help to explain some of those inexplicable miscarriages of yesteryear. One strain of infection, which you would never know was in your body, and which seems to be particularly important, is called Mycoplasma. We did not guess that this organism led to miscarriages until, in 1973, some controlled studies identified a subgroup called the "T strain" that showed up in woman after woman who was a recurrent spontaneous aborter.

The organism is a cross between a bacteria and a virus. It lives either in the vagina or in the man's genital tract and usually gives no symptoms. We request urine from both husband and wife in an unclean sample (by which I mean you are not asked to wash the area first), and a culture from the woman's cervix, and these are put together on a special growth plate. If Mycoplasma can be identified *before* you try for another pregnancy, we can treat it with antibiotics for 1 month, in both husband and wife. If you are already pregnant, then the treatment is much the same, except more care is taken in choosing the antibiotic used, so as not to harm the fetus; erythromycin is generally prescribed.

Another bacteria that may be implicated is Chlamydia, the "new VD," now about the most common sexually transmitted organism. Chlamydia may cause symptoms of pelvic infection, but you can also be a carrier and not know it. It is tested by taking a swab from within the cervix and then treated. Obviously it is preferable to have this infection identified before you try for another pregnancy. (Gonorrhea and syphilis, the other common venereal diseases, do not cause miscarriages, except in so much as they lead to generalized poor health.)

Toxoplasmosis is another well-known cause of miscarriages. We look for the organism in a blood test, by taking scrapings from the lining of the womb between pregnancies, or by testing menstrual blood with special antibody tests (see page 63).

Viruses are now assuming a more important role in the causation of miscarriages. Herpes simplex virus, or herpes (see pages 48–49), has been shown to have a very dramatic effect. If woman has herpes virus in the genital tract in the first 20 weeks of pregnancy, she has a three times higher chance of miscarrying than has the average woman. But the exact role of the herpes virus has not yet been determined. And there is no medication that will eradicate the virus from your body, only treatment to ease the discomfort.

I must emphasize that any infection, including the common ones such as Trichomonas and Monilia (thrush), may also be involved and should be treated. We still do not know what precise effect they have and how they cause miscarriages. More controlled studies have to be done on these common infections to draw really meaningful conclusions.

Talk of infections brings me to the subject of *intercourse in pregnancy*. There has been some recent work that shows intercourse may encourage infection of the fetus, placenta, amniotic membranes or amniotic fluid. These infections are introduced into the uterus by organisms carried on the backs of sperm and may lead to miscarriage, premature labor, or to amnionitis (see page 220). However, these findings are the result of a very recent study and have not yet been confirmed by other sources. I would not advise my patients against intercourse during pregnancy, for the risk of such infection is really very low.

You should, of course, practice the most careful hygiene whenever intercourse takes place, and, to be safe, if you have any history of miscarriages, I would advise avoiding full intercourse (by which I mean penetration of the penis into the vagina and ejaculation of sperm); though I would not advise against any other form of sexual activity that does not involve penetration. Take these precautions until past the time of your last miscarriage, particularly within the first 3 months of pregnancy. Later, there is not the same danger of infection, unless your cervix has already dilated and your obstetrician has said the membranes are showing—by which time your doctor will have warned you against intercourse anyway.

Chromosomal factors in the genetic makeup of the fetus (see pages 73–74) cause a great majority of early first miscarriages. There are a number of genetic causes, and if you have had *three* or more spontaneous miscarriages, you and your husband might consider genetics counseling to begin that form of investigation. Ideally, if you do miscarry at home, though this will be discomforting and unpleasant, you should keep the aborted fetus, collecting any tissue (gray substance among the clots of blood) in a clean container kept in the refrigerator, until you can get it to your doctor or to a genetics laboratory. Emotionally distressing though it may be, never throw away the product of a miscarriage at home; and do not put it in formalin, as this will negate the tests to be done.

With new improved techniques, geneticists can now look for chromosomal abnormalities in the aborted fetus. It may be discovered that the fetus has too few or too many chromosomes in its cells, or the chromosomes may have undergone structural changes (translocations) in which a fragment of one has become attached to the broken end of another. If any malformation of the chromosomes is found in one of your miscarriages, then the genetics counselor will be able to advise you of the risk to future pregnancies. There may be no genetic problem and you can try again without worry. You may be advised to try for another pregnancy and to have the fetus tested in the second trimester by amniocentesis, to see that it has not inherited any defects. (If it has, then you may choose to have a therapeutic abortion, to be spared giving birth to a defective baby.) If the prognosis is bad for both of you as parents, you might consider artificial insemination by donor (AID) or adoption.

Your doctor may also check out a new area of research in medicine: *immunology*. An enigma in the birth process has been fascinating the medical world for some years: the father supplies 50 percent of the fetus's tissues and these are foreign to the mother and should be rejected by her body just as an incompatible skin graft would be. There is, therefore, always the possibility that a recurrent spontaneous aborter is rejecting the father's tissue as part of the growing fetus. Mothers' bodies do not inherently reject their babies, and it is why they do *not* that has stimulated immunological research.

If we can learn why babies are usually not rejected, we may understand more about why some are. The theory at present is that something in the mother's blood circulation during pregnancy blocks the rejection process. This something is known as a "blocking antibody." Perhaps it is absent in some women who repeatedly miscarry. The level of blocking antibody can now be measured at a certain stage of pregnancy. Research is pursuing the possibility of remedying deficiencies. In the future medicine may include immunizing the mother against the father's tissue. But I must emphasize that this is all at the research stage. Do not expect your obstetrician to come up with the miracle drug to immunize you against such rejection.

Is anxiety or depression likely to mean you will miscarry?

The psychological aspects of pregnancy can be very important for recurrent aborters. I remember a midwife who worked with us who was pregnant herself and had suffered previous miscarriages. One day she delivered a woman's baby that was not well at birth. She went home and miscarried that night, possibly from a sense of her own failure in delivering another woman's child.

Recurrent aborters are usually very anxious. It is only natural if you have gone through one or more miscarriages to interpret every twinge or gas pain as the onset of premature labor. However, one positive outcome of this level of anxiety is that such women are likely to report any cramping or bleeding to their doctor as soon as it commences, so treatment can be introduced.

Examination and reassurance is often enough to settle the physical symptoms dramatically. From years of experience I know how emotionally trying repeated miscarriages can become. We recently interviewed thirty couples who had been recurrent aborters and we discovered negative feelings throughout their present pregnancies, both husband and wife suffering depression that they could not produce anything living. Husband blamed wife, and wife husband.

I have found that if you offer such patients a very positive attitude and ensure they get enough time and support from their doctor, you can frequently overcome what has turned into a "baby block." Reassurance, patience, and a willingness to listen to expressions of anxieties or problems can be a major source of healing. These couples are encouraged to attend our Pregnancy Support Clinic. They are seen every week, and the women are encouraged to stay in bed as much as possible and are given lots of emotional support, including a pregnancy "hot line" to their physician, nurse, or social worker.

Does bed rest really help? Some medical bodies still disparage the theory, but I believe that if you have suffered three or more consecutive spontaneous miscarriages, you will find extra bed rest does help. Scientifically it has been shown that lying in bed increases the blood supply to the placenta. Why it really works, we cannot be sure, but my advice is generally to stay in bed for a period extending 2 or 3 weeks beyond the last miscarriage (this will seldom mean any longer than 3 or 4 months). You may get up for meals and to go to the bathroom. But the more total the bed rest, the more beneficial.

Studies are being done that give some scientific support to the theory of bed rest. The effect of stress on certain hormones, such as adrenaline and cortisone, and their effects on pregnancy, are being looked into. There is only one piece of research in which psychotherapy was used with recurrent miscarriers, and the results showed a good progress rate. But we do not know whether these patients were put to bed as well as receiving the psychological support. Probably both factors are important. Further controlled studies are needed.

YOUR OWN HEALTH AND CONDITION

Operations and prescribed medications

If you have had a major operation under general anesthesia and some trauma to the body (caused by the surgery), I advise you to wait 6 months and then have a medical checkup to see if you are in general good health before trying to get pregnant.

If you have had extensive X rays beforehand, discuss this with your doctor.

If either husband or wife has had radioactive iodine treatment for a thyroid condition, wait at least a year before trying to get pregnant.

Therapies employing hormones such as synthetic progestogene are no longer used to diagnose pregnancies, since they can have a harmful effect on a fetus, similar to the effect of the Pill if you continue taking it once pregnant. So, if there is any chance of your becoming pregnant, avoid ingesting any form of hormone preparation.

As for the antibiotics that cause so many women anxiety—while it is true that tetracycline has been shown to stain the teeth of a baby a permanently greenish color, and that other antibiotics have various side effects, there are medications in this group that can be safely prescribed either during a pregnancy or if you feel you might be pregnant. If antibiotic therapy is necessary, your doctor will probably prescribe either penicillin, erythromycin, or one of the newer cephalosporins.

Over-the-counter medications

High-dose vitamins are very popular, particularly with the young and health-conscious. However, several of the individual vitamins taken in excess may well affect a fetus in pregnancy. So be careful about using excessive amounts of vitamins A, D, and C if there is any chance you might become pregnant (see page 127).

If you have been using diuretics to relieve premenstrual soreness of the breasts, you must take care during the second half of your cycle if you should get pregnant, as diuretics have been proved harmful to a fetus.

Antithyroid medications may affect the newborn and should not be taken if you are trying to get pregnant. Some are better than others, however, and if this becomes a problem to you, have your doctor adjust the dosage and the type taken so that you can feel safe about a future pregnancy.

Do not take any aspirin (or medications that include aspirin), if you think you might be pregnant. Midline body defects such as harelip and cleft palate have been attributed to this drug. If you really have to use any aspirinlike drug, I advise you to use Tylenol. But, if you did take aspirin in early pregnancy, before conception was confirmed, do not worry. It is very common to have taken some aspirin when pregnant and harmful effects are extremely rare. If you are on maintenance aspirin for heart or joint disease, discuss this with your specialist before you get pregnant.

Be cautious in your use of the most common over-the-counter medications such as cold remedies, antacids, and iron tablets. All of them have come under suspicion and, especially if taken in high doses, might cause some harm to a fetus during the period of organogenesis. Ask your doctor's advice on what you may or may not use.

Social drugs

I am referring in this section to all forms of relaxing, entertaining, and mind-expanding drugs, many of which are used quite widely these days. I appreciate that there is little use in my taking a didactic, old-fashioned approach and saying "Don't use any drug, ever, for social reasons, because they are all bad for you, and for the pregnancy." But I do want to take the opportunity to put down some hard facts that have emerged from recent research, which should help you firm up your resolve and make your own judgments.

The main difficulty with judging the effect of any social drug on an average pregnancy, or the state of a woman's health before pregnancy, is that most of the research has been done on those who take the drug to extremes: chronic or addicted users. These are the people who come to the clinics for help and who are available for research projects. They often take multiple drugs or have diet deficiencies that may also affect their health. How the more conservative usage that is typical of the average person affects a pregnancy is much harder to deduce and has not in fact been reported. The necessary studies are almost impossible to make. All I can do, however, is make my own assessment of the research that is available and give you a sort of precautionary overview.

Many women on narcotics do not ovulate and do not even conceive. Doctors can tell by urine screening tests if patients are on narcotics and which kind. Fifty percent of infants of drug abusers have complications at birth resulting from withdrawal symptoms.

ALCOHOL

The effects of drinking on pregnancy are now quite well established, and urgent calls to pregnant women to severely curtail their drinking have been going out very recently, heavily supported by the efforts of the March of Dimes. If you are an alcoholic, or are indulging in a life style of which heavy drinking is a part, you do run the risk of harming a potential baby.

How harmful is drinking? Since so many women ask me how much is too much, I think it is time to set some limits. An alcoholic is a person who suffers withdrawal symptoms if she does not drink. She drinks in excess of six stiff drinks a day (at least one bottle of hard liquor), or about two bottles of wine, or more than twelve beers. An alcoholic also tends to drink early in the morning and most of the day. If you feel you may be an alcoholic, I advise you to seek help for that condition *before* becoming pregnant, as the serious consequences for a baby are sufficient to warrant a therapeutic abortion should you conceive.

Alcoholics run the risk of giving their baby fetal alcohol syndrome, a recognizable pattern of both physical and mental defects. The baby is more likely to be of low birth weight (making survival harder) and to have a much smaller head size than normal. These children never catch up on normal growth and are usually mentally deficient, because of their smaller brain size. They also tend to suffer from conditions that will be disturbing throughout life: they may be jittery and badly coordinated, with short attention spans and serious behavioral problems. As there are reportedly at least 1 million women alcoholics in America of childbearing age, the problem is particularly acute among groups of teenagers, where drinking to excess is often a big problem.

But what about normal drinking? Is there a safe limit? Right now, the official government advice on how much alcohol is advisable during pregnancy is—"complete abstinence." The U.S. surgeon general came out with a statement in Washington in July 1981, advising doctors to recommend that expectant mothers have *no* alcohol at all. The reason for this urgent appeal to women to stop drinking is that, from all the research work available, it still is not clear whether there is *no* danger in just 1 ounce of alcohol (a couple of drinks) or whether the danger is cumulative and does not take effect unless you are drinking more than 3 ounces of pure alcohol a day (about one full bottle of wine).

If you are contemplating a pregnancy, do you have to go on the wagon before conceiving? How long will it take to "dry out"?

As I have said, alcoholics should seek proper treatment before conceiving. For the normal drinker, there is no need to "dry out" for any length of time before a pregnancy. Just be very careful around the time you might conceive, during that dangerous period when the embryo is forming (the first 12 weeks) and its brain and nervous system, particularly, are developing.

When you are pregnant, be prepared to *attempt* to cut out all drinking. If you are only a light or weekend drinker anyway, it may be easy to give up even that small amount. If you must, limit yourself to one very light drink on the weekend. If you find such abstinence impossible, and you feel left out in the company of your husband or friends, add a drop of wine or spirits to mineral water, seltzer, soda, or whatever mixer you are used to, and permit yourself an extremely watered-down mixed drink, preferably a long one.

Pregnancy can be a trying time for some couples' relationships. The husband may begin to feel his wife is no longer interested in him, no longer sexually outgoing and, on top of all that, if his usually daredevil, fun-loving partner turns nunlike and sober on him, then he may well feel parenthood is creating a change in life style he does not altogether welcome.

CIGARETTES

Cigarettes are seldom viewed by smokers as a form of drug abuse, but they are as strong and powerful a drug as any mentioned in this section. The fact that their use is legal is a matter of politics, rather than of medical ethics. The truth is that cigarette smoking has been found, in report after report, to have a potentially harmful effect on the unborn child.

The toxic effect of smoking in pregnancy has been noted since the late 1950s, when the incidence of premature low-birth-weight babies born to smokers was first understood. By low birth weight, I mean up to 1 pound lighter than full-term babies born to nonsmokers. The survival chances of a low-birth-weight baby are significantly lower than normal. Smoking also appears to be responsible for a higher proportion of babies who die in the uterus, spontaneously abort, or die within a week of birth. Nearly 10 years ago, the U.S. surgeon general estimated that cigarette smoking was responsible for 5 percent of all perinatal deaths. It is probable that smoke inhalation deprives the mother's blood of much capacity to carry oxygen to the developing fetus.

Do you have to give up smoking before you get pregnant? I am sure it would be better if you gave it up altogether, for your continuing good health aside from pregnancy. But being realistic, I know that quitting smoking can cause great problems for the chronic smoker. There is some evidence that if you can give up cigarettes by the fourth month of pregnancy, you have a better chance of producing a normal, healthy baby. The worst risk to the fetus may be in the fourth month. If you can minimize the number you smoke, that will help. For example, if you smoke *less* than a pack a day, the risk of a perinatal death, abruption (separation) of the placenta, or low-birth-weight baby is increased by 22 percent; if you smoke *more* than a pack a day, the risk is increased by 44 percent. But, if you smoke fewer than four cigarettes a day, the risk drops considerably.

There is conflicting evidence that if you have been a smoker for years, and have given it up for the pregnancy, it will still have a harmful effect on your baby. Certain evidence even shows that if you stand in a room with someone else who is smoking it could affect *your* baby. Ideally, I suggest you and your husband both stop smoking a year before trying to conceive. And, once you suspect you are pregnant, you should keep out of crowded smoky parties or bars, and sit in nonsmoking sections of planes and trains. Fortunately, most women (even many smokers) loathe the smell of cigarette smoke in the first trimester of pregnancy.

MARIJUANA

Like alcohol, marijuana is very commonly used as a sexual stimulant, and many women become pregnant while they have been smoking some form of cannabis. But does marijuana actually cause birth defects? Many women patients have asked me this question. Marijuana smoking has become part of an accepted life style, not only among the poor but among the affluent educated and sophisticated.

If you and your husband have been moderate (not chronic—by which I mean constant daily use) smokers of marijuana for several years before you plan a pregnancy, there is no research to show that this will cause any harmful effect on your baby. However, from the latest report issued by the Public Health Service (National Institute on Drug Abuse), the most obvious effect you may notice *before* pregnancy is a difficulty in conceiving.

Marijuana smoking in men appears to lower the level of the reproductive hormones, so there is less testosterone in the system. It also temporarily decreases the sperm count and sperm motility, and has been shown to increase the number of abnormal sperm. Women have not been tested as thoroughly as men, but there is reason to believe that too much marijuana can increase the number of menstrual cycles during which ovulation does not take place, or can cause ovulation without adequate corpus luteum action (see page 89). If you are having any problems conceiving, maybe it is time to stop smoking marijuana now. The drug may be encouraging your sexual activity, but it also may be discouraging reproductive activity.

Once you are pregnant, I do not believe you should smoke marijuana, even occasionally. There is no evidence to show that it causes fetal malformations, but the chemicals within the drug have not yet been thoroughly tested. There is some proof that it can lead to low-birth-weight babies, whose chances of survival and normal health are initially less than those of normal-birth-weight babies. It will not have this effect on the fetus if you smoked it in the past but have already stopped—so that should not worry you.

COCAINE

Cocaine may be a fashionable drug in certain quarters, but it is a dangerous drug that, especially if used in excess, can be harmful to your health. Any research that has been conducted on the effects of cocaine has been on addicts or habitual users and so we really have no conclusive evidence about its effect on the occasional user who wants to know if she may "snort" the drug at parties, or other special occasions, even though she is pregnant.

Basically, if you are pregnant or there is a chance you might be pregnant, you should discontinue use of cocaine. As long as you have not been an habitual user, your system will not be full of the drug, so there is unlikely to be any long-term effect on your baby from *past* usage.

Although the effect of cocaine on the fetus has not been re-corded, the effect it has on you will be transmitted many times more strongly to the baby. Cocaine use during pregnancy will probably increase the risk of a low-birth-weight baby, or even a miscarriage. Cocaine is associated with environmental risks such as broken body rhythms, insomnia, and poor eating hab-its—and many cocaine users take other, softer drugs as well—all of which is bad for your own health and for the pregnancy.

"SPEED" AND OTHER AMPHETAMINES

All amphetamines are dangerous drugs that must not be used in pregnancy or in the second half of a menstrual cycle in which you might become pregnant. Speed increases the risk of having a low-birth-weight baby and of premature labor. The poor diet and insomnia that accompanies the habitual use of speed will make your general health weak and the pregnancy unsafe. I advise you to stop taking such drugs at least a month before trying to conceive and never take them if you might be, or are, pregnant. There is no evidence to show that a past history of their use will have any effect on future childbearing, so long as you have since changed your life style, eat well, rest, and exercise regularly. In fact, affluent teenagers who have recently fallen into a bad life style, with drugs and irregular habits, have been shown to fare better in pregnancy than young people who have always lived in poverty; because their years of careful home life and adequate nutrition have protected their bodies to some degree.

LSD

Findings on the effect of the use of this drug before pregnancy are more complex. There used to be talk that by merely taking LSD a few times in youth, you could affect your chromosomes adversely and consequently give birth to a baby with some birth defects. Since the widespread use of LSD by young people in the late sixties and early seventies, however, that generation has begun to reproduce and we have not noted an increase in birth defects in the babies of parents who experimented during that period with LSD to a small degree. So do not panic if your history includes some experimentation with LSD. But do advise your doctor about it when you become pregnant. Your doctor will not be shocked; it is not the role of the physician to be judgmental.

If you are concerned because you used a substantial quantity of LSD in the past, or have been using it recently, then do let your doctor know of this anxiety before a pregnancy. He or she might suggest you go to a genetics center for chromosomal testing. If that would reassure you, then I suggest that you and your husband (if he has taken LSD, the danger to his chromosomes will be the same as to yours) seriously consider such an evaluation—even though it may be costly.

Otherwise the dangers of LSD are seen more in the accompanying poor life style, diet low in nutrition and high in junk foods, and in the hidden dangers of whatever has been mixed with it if it was bought off the streets.

Once there is any chance you might be pregnant, or if you are pregnant, never use LSD. It is a dangerous and illegal drug and not worth the potential risk to your child's health and happiness, or to your own.

HOW LONG SHOULD YOU HAVE STOPPED TAKING HARD DRUGS BEFORE YOU TRY TO CONCEIVE?

If you have been addicted to a drug such as heroin or cocaine, you should be free from the habit by at least 1 year before trying to conceive. To ensure that you are in general good health, I suggest you have a full physical checkup, including tests of your liver function. To overcome the harmful effects of addiction in the year before conception, good nutrition and plenty of sleep and relaxation are essential. Your past will not have a long-term harmful effect on your future childbearing as long as you are clean of hard drugs, and are not tempted to substitute with other "soft" ones.

Many former heroin addicts, now in methadone maintenance programs, give birth to normal, healthy babies. They must be attending proper methadone maintenance clinics that are prepared to offer full pregnancy support management with the cooperation of their obstetrician. Their dosage will be altered throughout the pregnancy; and also during the period of nursing to minimize the methadone content in the mother's milk.

It goes without saying that it would be better if all women were clear of heroin and methadone and other such drugs before they became pregnant, but that is sadly not a very realistic hope these days in our major cities. Babies born to women who are currently heroin addicts are born addicted and suffer withdrawal symptoms at birth. Drug addiction in the newborn baby is a difficult and distressing condition to treat and it can easily lead to death.

CURRENT MEDICAL CONDITIONS

Can you get pregnant if you have . . . ?

EPILEPSY

These days women who suffer from epilepsy (about 1 percent of the female population) are controlled on anticonvulsant drugs. Epilepsy does not affect fertility, and there is no reason why an epileptic woman should not contemplate pregnancy, although it will have to be specially managed to avoid minor complications.

During pregnancy, half of those with epilepsy will not have any more seizures than normal. But there are some women whose condition does deteriorate (less than 30 percent of all epileptic women) and they have to be specially cared for. Vomiting in early pregnancy can become a problem, too, for epileptic women, if it results in a smaller amount of their anticonvulsant medications being absorbed and leads to an increase in the convulsions.

Most anticonvulsant drugs, in themselves, will not be harmful to the pregnancy, but they can lead to a deficiency of folic acid, a vitamin that is necessary for the baby's tissue growth. So any epileptic woman on anticonvulsant drugs should take a vitamin supplement containing folic acid to prevent the resulting anemia. (In Britain, iron and folic acid are prescribed to all pregnant women in a combined tablet, as the folic acid helps the iron become absorbed, thus preventing anemia. In the U.S., maternal vitamin supplements usually contain both iron and folic acid.)

As some anticonvulsant drugs have been linked with congenital birth defects, it is important to see your doctor before becoming pregnant, to discuss the treatment of your condition. If medication is still required to prevent the seizures, you should continue to use some form of medication. Phenobarbital is the safest of the drugs for use before conceiving and, if possible, for the first trimester (the period of organogenesis). In more severe cases, phenytoin, the other common anticonvulsant, could be used—but it is best not to take it until the second trimester. But if your seizures are very bad, lasting 2 to 3 minutes, they themselves could damage the baby, and phenytoin, the stronger drug, would probably be the safer alternative.

With careful supervision by your obstetrician and your epilepsy physician, you should have a normal, happy pregnancy and birth.

DIABETES

There is no longer any maternal mortality associated with diabetes, which is an incredible advance since only recently. Before 1922, when a Canadian doctor discovered the hormone insulin, few young adults or children with the disease lived long enough to have children. A diabetic woman was seldom healthy enough to marry and have children. In the last 10 years, however, exciting changes have occurred. A lot of research has been completed in this field, and plans of management have been outlined in large medical schools to guide obstetricians. Now a diabetic woman need not fear she cannot have a baby.

Oral diabetes medications have been implicated in causing fetal abnormalities. These medications have now been largely replaced by insulin injections or careful diet control. So, if you are taking oral drugs for diabetes and are considering becoming pregnant, see your physician now and you may be switched to diet control or to insulin injections. These injections are safe before or during pregnancy.

Let me stress that, although pregnancy is safe for the diabetic, you are going to need careful management from the very beginning. In fact, I believe it is a good idea for you to keep a basal body temperature chart at all times, so that you can detect a possible pregnancy at a very early stage—particularly if your periods are irregular. Then you will be able to tell your doctor as soon as you *think* you are pregnant.

If you are a chronic sufferer of diabetes, you must make sure to attend a special pregnancy clinic, preferably in a large teaching hospital. Your condition will probably have to be managed by a select group of physicians and nutritional counselors, skilled not only in the treatment of diabetes but in this particular form of obstetrics; not all doctors will have this specialized knowledge. Should you live far from such a hospital, you may have to be hospitalized for some of your pregnancy. But if you act wisely now, the outcome of that pregnancy should be fine and happy.

HEART DISEASE

Some 1 percent of pregnant women today have some form of heart disease. Even though their pregnancies may not be as simple as those of other women, most women with congenital heart disease, including some cardiac patients who have valves implanted, are now successfully giving birth to healthy babies. Some more serious cases may have to be hospitalized for the whole of their pregnancy, and for a period afterward.

If you are a woman with a heart condition, and contemplate getting pregnant, you must seek your doctor's advice beforehand. Your cardiologist will be able to assess your heart's capacity for the increased load and strain the pregnancy will bring. So much more is now understood about the changes in the mother's heart and vascular system during pregnancy, that a confident assessment can be made beforehand. The days when heart disease in a woman required therapeutic abortion or sterilization are over.

If your cardiologist gives permission for a pregnancy and does not think you will have to be hospitalized for the full term, be prepared nevertheless for restrictions on physical activity, and for lots of bed rest. Certain medications may have to be modified, particularly if you take anticoagulants. If you are receiving injections of heparin, which is the main drug used, it is considered safe to continue them in pregnancy. The oral drugs,

however, have caused some controversy, and have been implicated in causing fetal abnormalities or bleeding. These may have
to be discontinued.

Drugs used to alter the rate of the heartbeat, such as quini-
dine and propranolol, may both be used under supervision as
safe for the baby. In some instances, however, after use of propranolol, the newborn shows some temporary distress at birth
(such as respiratory depression), but this is not long-lasting and
should not cause you to panic. Digitalis, which is widely used,
has not been shown to have any harmful effects in pregnancy,
and may be used if indicated.

Because of the importance of preventing infections, some
heart patients are given antibiotics at the time of delivery. But
again, that is not a cause for concern, as safe antibiotics are
available and often given at the deliveries of high-risk patients.

The only warning to women with severe heart disease is that
sometimes the effects of their disease can reduce the amount
of oxygen supplied to the baby, which can lead to an increased
incidence of spontaneous abortion, premature labor, and occasionally to death of the baby in the uterus. I mention this so
that you will not be too disappointed if a pregnancy ends this
way for you. If your doctor gives you the go-ahead, you may
try again to conceive—only this time with even more careful
management by your physician.

ASTHMA

Just under 3 percent of the American population has asthma,
and its incidence as a disease of pregnancy is 0.6 percent. If
you are asthmatic, there is no reason to be concerned about
the outcome of your pregnancy.

Because of the chemical changes in the pregnant woman, we
used to think that asthma improved in pregnancy. But this is
an unpredictable side effect. Some women improve, but in most
the asthma stays about the same as in their nonpregnant state.
The great majority of asthmatic women go through pregnancy

and deliver quite normally, though severe asthmatics will need very careful management, particularly toward the end of the pregnancy.

Your baby will have a 5 percent chance of developing the disease early in life, with a greater risk if both you and your husband are asthmatics and an increasing risk as your child gets older.

There are many different asthma medications available. If you might be pregnant, it is important not to use any of them without first consulting your doctor. (I hope you will seek his or her advice even before becoming pregnant.) The treatment you are taking might do your baby more harm than the good it is doing you. *Any* drug containing iodide must not be taken if you could be pregnant, as it goes through the placenta and can damage the fetal thyroid. Cortisone may be used for severe attacks of asthma, just as if you were not pregnant. There is no evidence linking this drug with any fetal abnormalities, if it is used in the short term.

CANCER

If you have been treated for any malignant condition and are contemplating a pregnancy, you must discuss it with your specialist. There is much more medical information now available and new tests that can be done to see if various types of cancer might recur or flare up during a pregnancy. The chances of your being able to have a normal happy pregnancy and delivery are very high.

THYROID DISEASE

A thyroid sufferer on therapy will probably need some form of adjustment to the medication being used. If you are contemplating a pregnancy, do consult a doctor before you conceive, as radioactive tests or thyroid therapy are dangerous, will cross the placenta, and can harm the fetus.

HIGH BLOOD PRESSURE

During pregnancy, high blood pressure can present potential problems, which is why obstetricians regularly check women's blood pressure at each visit. If you are hypertensive and are contemplating a pregnancy, see your doctor now to stabilize the condition, adjust the drugs used, and begin investigations to determine the cause. Such tests are much easier to do when you are not pregnant.

In about one third of patients with high blood pressure the cause is never found. The condition is then known as "essential hypertension." Even then the prognosis for a successful pregnancy is good. You will be treated exactly as you were when not pregnant. Antihypertensive drugs are available that will not harm the baby.

The danger of high blood pressure is that you may get a superimposed condition known as pre-eclamptic toxemia, which complicates about 10 percent of pregnancies in America and which is a concern to all obstetricians. Pre-eclampsia can only happen in pregnancy, not before hand (see page 114).

GERMAN MEASLES (RUBELLA)

German measles can be a very serious disease in pregnancy. If you develop the infection in the early stages of pregnancy it can lead to severe fetal abnormalities (these occur in as many as 50 percent of such pregnancies). Even if you contract German measles in the third trimester, your baby can still be affected, though the probability is far lower.

The connection between German measles and fetal abnormalities was discovered in 1941 by an Australian doctor who noticed that babies with severe eye defects were born to mothers exposed to the infection. It was some years, however, before the medical world accepted the link. Since 1969, rubella vaccines have been available. The recommendation is that you have a blood test to see if you are immune to German measles *before* you get pregnant. If you are not already immune (you had the disease in childhood or contact with the infection), you should then be vaccinated. It is *essential* that for the following 3 months you avoid conception. You must not conceive when there is any of the vaccine in your body, as it is a live, though weakened, virus. Fortunately, today in America and Britain, most children are immunized before they are ten, and so most young women are immune when they become pregnant.

There are minor side effects to the vaccination (the incidence is about 10 percent). Some patients experience temporary arthritic pains. But the success rate of the vaccine is 95 percent.

If you know that you were vaccinated in the past and are now contemplating a pregnancy, I would advise you still be tested for immunity before becoming pregnant. We do not know how long-lasting the effect of the vaccine is. The natural disease, however, has an almost permanent protective effect against recurrence.

YOUR SEXUAL HISTORY

A *past history of promiscuity worries you*

Despite any feelings of guilt you may have, there is no reason why previous promiscuous behavior should have any effect on a future pregnancy, unless it resulted in a disease that caused structural damage to your genital region. I know that some women feel they will be punished for their prior sexual conduct by being unable to give birth to a normal, healthy baby. Well, no such punishment exists in the medical world. All I can say is, do not indulge in promiscuous behavior once you have decided to get pregnant, or once there is any chance you may be pregnant. I say that not as a moralist, but merely from the protective standpoint. You do not want to contract venereal disease or herpes once pregnant—as treatment is very hard after conception, and there may be fetal effects.

If you have any deep concerns or anxieties that may in fact be hindering your happiness or fertility, go to your gynecologist. You should have an internal examination and be screened for venereal disease and vaginal infection. Put your mind and your conscience at rest.

Past or current VD or herpes: What can be done?

Gonorrhea is the most significant of the venereal diseases, because if you contract it in the vagina or cervix, there is a 15 percent chance of its spreading to the Fallopian tubes, which could leave you sterile. If you have gonorrhea in pregnancy, it can harm the baby's eyes during the process of delivery. (The bacteria may reach the baby before birth, when the water breaks.) However, all babies receive eye medication at birth to prevent eye damage from the gonococcus or other bacteria present in the vagina.

So, if there is any danger of your having contracted gonorrhea in the past, and you have not been screened for it, do check with your doctor before you try to get pregnant. Symptoms usually appear 2 to 8 days after contact. A man may see a whitish-yellow discharge from his penis, feel itching or burning when urinating. A woman may have burning urination, vaginal discharge, or fever and stomach pain. In some cases neither the man nor the woman will have any symptoms.

At the first pregnancy visit your doctor will test for gonorrhea by taking a culture from the cervical smear. If there is any history of exposure to, or of treatment for, gonorrhea in your past, you should be checked again before getting pregnant. If you have been having a vaginal discharge or any bladder symptoms, then you should ask to be screened *before* pregnancy. If you practice rectal or oral sex, you must tell your doctor, for these areas should be examined for the infection too.

The treatment for gonorrhea is with penicillin, which is safe during pregnancy. It is advisable to be medically clear of any venereal infection before becoming pregnant. If screening shows you have gonorrhea, then your husband, or partner, will also be treated. At the time of the gonorrhea screening, you will also be given a blood test for syphilis, to ascertain that you are free of all VDs.

Syphilis is now quite infrequent during pregnancy in America, as any couple contemplating marriage is automatically screened for it before their license is issued. This is a mammoth screening of the whole population, in an attempt to wipe out the disease. But if you do contract syphilis and know nothing about it (it can be asymptomatic), and if it goes untreated for long, it may affect your internal organs and lead to general deterioration of your health. Worse, if you become pregnant not knowing you have syphilis, the spirochete can cross the placenta and cause harm to the fetus in several ways: from minor congenital abnormalities to death in the uterus before birth.

The most common screening test for syphilis is the VDRL (Veneral Disease Research Laboratory test.) It is not specific for syphilis, so if a positive result is obtained you will need further testing before any treatment is given. All pregnant women are screened at the time of their first pregnancy visit because of the serious effects syphilis can have on a baby. If you have any known history of syphilis, you should be screened before getting pregnant to make sure you are clear of the disease. Once treated before a pregnancy, there is no chance of the previous infection affecting your baby.

Herpes. Genital herpes simplex virus is a venereal disease that is becoming increasingly common in America, particularly in major urban areas, where it can be said to have reached epidemic proportions, overtaking gonorrhea as the most common sexually transmitted disease. It can be transmitted by intercourse or by oral sex.

The virus lies dormant in nerve tissue and is resistant to

medication, and unfortunately there is as yet no treatment that has proved effective in eradicating it from the body. If genital herpes is contracted before pregnancy, it will not necessarily lead to a recurrence in pregnancy, although nothing can be done at the present time to prevent possible flare-ups.

Treatment is symptomatic and is usually in the form of anesthetic ointment to ease the pain and discomfort. As this is a virus, not a bacteria, antibiotics will not eradicate it. The lesions may be vaporized with a laser beam, but again this is not curative.

The main effect of herpes is an increase in the rate of spontaneous miscarriage in early pregnancy, and it may, very rarely, cause congenital abnormalities in the fetus. The worst effect it seems to have is that the baby has a 50 percent chance of contracting the infection during vaginal delivery if the virus is present in the genital tract. If you have a history of herpes, tell your doctor about it, even if there are no symptoms (that is, lesions in the genital area) when you conceive. He or she will take routine cultures from the cervix and labia during your pregnancy. If the virus is present in the cervix or vagina in the last trimester, your obstetrician will probably advise birth by caesarean section. With the performance of a caesarean section, you can be relieved to know the baby is unlikely to contract herpes.

Trichomonal vaginitis is a common sexually transmitted infection that itself has no harmful effect on a pregnancy since it remains localized to the vagina. The problem here is that metronidazole, the drug normally prescribed for treatment, should not be used during the first trimester of pregnancy. (It has been proved to have bad effects on the fetuses of mice.) Even in late pregnancy, it should be used only in the most severe cases. If you do have a vaginal discharge, it is essential to get it cleared up before you become pregnant, so that the treatment may be prescribed without problem. Once treated successfully, the effects of the drug will not harm a future pregnancy.

Monilia, *fungal vaginitis*, or *thrush* are synonymous. The incidence of thrush increases in pregnancy and it is a common complaint. The chemical balance of the vagina becomes more acid, encouraging the growth of the fungus. It is not a venereally transmitted disease in the true sense of the term. The organism may normally live in the vagina, but is kept in check by bacteria. Pregnancy, or antibiotic therapy, can disturb this balance. The fungus may also be transmitted to your husband or partner, producing a dry scaly rash on his penis, so treatment is often necessary for both of you.

In pregnancy, the problem with thrush is if you are still infected at the time of going into labor, for it may affect the baby's mouth on its passage through the vagina. It may also cause poor healing of your episiotomy. It is, therefore, advisable to have the discharge treated before pregnancy, or early in the pregnancy, with nystatin—which is safe for use after conception.

Condyloma acuminatum is the medical name for warts in the vaginal or labial area. They usually have no effect on a pregnancy, except that they can enlarge and then may cause problems with delivery due to obstruction, or get in the way of an episiotomy. If you have any warts in the perineal area you should have them removed before you get pregnant as podophyllin, the prescribed medication, is not allowed during pregnancy.

YOUR LIFE STYLE

Exercise

Exercise is not a problem in a healthy pregnancy. In the last 15 years, everyone's attitudes on this subject have changed dramatically. In your mother's day, a woman was persuaded to sit down and put her feet up from the moment she coyly told her husband about the expected baby. These days, however, your husband or doctor should not be surprised if you continue with your daily or weekly tennis game, jog 2 miles a day, ride the crowded subway to and from work right through most of your pregnancy, or commute 30 miles a day behind the wheel of a car.

Generally speaking, my attitude is that as long as you are healthy, and everything goes well with the pregnancy, you can live your life as you used to. (I do not give the same advice to anyone who has had more than one spontaneous abortion or who has bleeding or cramping early in pregnancy. See page 102.) Be just as active and involved in the outside world, so long as you remember to get extra rest, eat well, and be sure to get a proper night's sleep throughout. Do not overtire yourself, for your reserves will be down and it will take longer to recuperate. (No quick half-hour rest resuscitates an exhausted pregnant woman. It may take a day or more to get back to normal.)

The only time you should *possibly* be careful not to overdo the level of your exercises is actually guarded by nature herself. In the first trimester (12 weeks) of pregnancy, when too much exertion may well rob the growing embryo of valuable oxygen for its development, you may feel far too exhausted or unwell (from nausea or vomiting associated with the first 12 weeks) to want to participate in regular exercise or sports. So, fatigue is your own limiting factor, dictating your life style in this crucial period—rather than leaving it up to individual common sense or judgment.

There is evidence to show that the extra bed rest your body forces upon you at this time increases the blood supply to the fetus, thereby supplying it with more of the oxygen vital to its development. Many women feel so drowsy that they say they could fall asleep standing up—or walking down the street. One patient of mine, an avid runner and calisthenics fan, felt *guilty* about her drowsiness and thought she was letting herself down by not attending exercise classes for those 3 months. I assured her that her stamina and vigor would return once the nausea and sleepiness waned after the end of the first trimester—and sure enough they did. She found herself running and exercising quite happily until the end of her sixth month of pregnancy.

Can you harm a baby by too much sport?

Some recent books have pointed out some female sporting achievements during pregnancy that I feel deserve a mention. If you are worrying that your life is going to change, making you dull and sedentary after you have had a baby, or while you are pregnant, just read what some stalwart women have accomplished: June Irwin was 3½ months pregnant when she won a bronze medal for platform diving in the 1952 Summer Olympics. Andrea Mead Lawrence was in her first trimester of pregnancy when she won two gold medals for alpine racing in the 1952 Winter Olympics. Wendy Boglioli, Olympic track champion, was in her fifth month of pregnancy when she competed in the 100-yards freestyle in 1978. And Mary Jones was near the end of her eighth month of pregnancy when she ran the 13.1-mile Dallas White Rock Marathon in December 1976, in 2 hours and 5 minutes. (*Womanlist*, Atheneum, 1981.)

Personally, I do *not* recommend that you undertake either alpine racing or platform diving in pregnancy, and these feats I have quoted are obviously those of the rare compulsive sportswomen who will not give up competition for anything. As a rule, I would say by all means continue with your favorite sport, but not at a competitive level. Competition forces you to take risks, with your own life and with that of the fetus. Both Margaret Court and Evonne Goolagong, world tennis champions, played tennis right through their pregnancies, but not at competition level. They kept up their expertise, fitness, and self-confidence by playing "friendly" matches.

Horseback riding is another sport that I would not encourage a pregnant woman to undertake. Mainly because the risk of falling is too great. Britain's Princess Anne, however, refused to give up horseback riding during her two pregnancies. And Mary Bacon, a professional woman jockey who has ridden more than 300 winners, one day rode three consecutive races and then went to the hospital to give birth to her daughter. Again, she is hardly the average woman, and you do not have to feel a sense of failure if you cannot top her achievement. If you are a committed horseback rider and feel your horse would perish from lack of affection and attention during the 9 months of your pregnancy, then ride gently, taking few risks.

Marathon running should not be undertaken in pregnancy, as the *prolonged* rise in body temperature may have the potential to harm the developing fetus. Jogging should be restricted to 20 minutes at a time.

Will too much exercise make it hard to conceive?

No one really knows the scientific answer to this question, which is why you may read conflicting reports on the subject. I have seen some feminist books recently quoting the evidence of G. D. Erdelyi, who surveyed 729 women athletes in 1962 and found that none was prevented from menstruating by her athletics. But that is not evidence enough to provide all the information. I have seen patients who have suffered spells of amenorrhea (lack of menstrual periods) when they have been in training for something as strenuous as the New York Marathon. Such high levels of training, and the physical overload, put a burden on the body and cause the hormonal balance to compensate. Very high levels of exercise and training can make the body produce excess testosterone, which in itself is a masculinizing hormone (see page 36) and can hinder the female reproductive hormones.

Usually temporary amenorrhea clears up after a few months

of more restful life. But I have also seen professional dancers—particularly young ballerinas who are compulsive about their work and exercise routines and are so thin as to be near-starved—who suffer acute amenorrhea and consequently become infertile.

If you are having a problem conceiving and feel your lack of periods may be due to your level of fitness, sportswomanship, or weight, then why not try a long vacation, with no workouts, and see if your body adjusts naturally?

Will having a child affect you in the future as a sportswoman?

Many women still suffer from believing the myth that once they have become mothers they will go into a physical decline. However, there seems to be some evidence that, once you have given birth (or been pregnant nearly to term) your hormones adjust themselves to an easier harmony; anxiety levels often diminish and, with a more emotionally full (if not fulfilled!) life, you may find your sense of self-confidence is greatly increased, so enabling you to perform better on the field, the track, or in the boardroom.

How can you be sure exercise or dancing will not bring on a miscarriage?

Let me emphasize that there are certain women who should *not* exercise vigorously during pregnancy. Anyone who has suffered more than one spontaneous miscarriage, who has bleeding early in pregnancy, or any cramping, should be discouraged from exercising above the moderate level. Repeat spontaneous aborters who have been recommended complete bed rest until they get past the point of their last miscarriage should not exercise at all. But unless your doctor specifically states that because of your medical history or condition you should avoid any form of exercise, you can feel confident that jumping up and down, throwing your arms over your head, touching your toes, twisting to the left or right, will not bring on any problems.

Are there any prohibitions?

If squash and racquetball are your games, I suggest you take up tennis, swimming, running, or special pregnancy exercise classes for these few months of your life to keep you in shape. Sports that involve sudden bursts of excess energy *might* provoke a miscarriage, particularly in early pregnancy.

Do you have to exercise in pregnancy?

The answer is yes, I really do feel you should take some form of exercise. Pregnancy can be a time of laziness (and overeating) if you are not careful. You will begin to feel very self-indulgent and emotionally introverted as the developing fetus becomes more real to you with the passing months. To encourage a healthy diet and a healthy pregnancy, I advise you to do at least a lot of walking, on a daily basis, even if running, tennis, or swimming are not your custom. You should not be sitting on silk cushions eating chocolates, even if you feel like doing nothing else. Good circulation, strong muscles, and a sound cardiovascular system will make pregnancy and labor a happier, easier time for both you and the baby. So even if you have never exercised before, make pregnancy the time to begin a personal fitness program.

TRAVEL

Is travel a mistake if you are planning to get pregnant?

If you are planning a major trip, or an extensive tour abroad, seize the time for it now, before a pregnancy. Once you are pregnant, there will be many considerations before deciding whether travel is all right. For example, a really extensive trip can be ruined in the first trimester of a pregnancy by possible nausea and excessive sleepiness. Moreover, air travel may be contraindicated in the early months of pregnancy if your doctor feels there is any risk of miscarriage. In the final trimester of pregnancy, most airlines will accept you as a passenger up to 4 weeks before delivery date, though you may have to provide a doctor's note (if you are in your eighth month or more) declaring you are fit to travel. As Pan Am and other major airlines say, they do not want to be held responsible for your medical condition on board. (For further information on travel in pregnancy, see pages 150–151.)

One more word on travel before pregnancy. Many couples who have been having difficulties conceiving during workaday life find they achieve conception while they are on vacation or away on a business trip. The relaxation and enforced intimacy that come with new surroundings and a change from the humdrum, too-hectic routine can be the magic wand you prayed for. In many instances, therefore, travel can be a decided boost before a pregnancy.

WORK

Is it harmful to the baby if you hold a full-time job during pregnancy?

Since the days when your mother was carrying you, one of the biggest revolutions has been in the numbers of women in full-time employment who remain employed throughout pregnancy and after childbirth. Countless women have worked until the day they go into labor, with no apparent effect on the health of the baby they deliver.

I do not believe that work, in itself, can have any harmful

effect on a fetus; indeed, I expect that the outside occupation, interest of co-workers, and opportunity to discuss the impending birth with other women are of more value to pregnancy than previous generations ever imagined.

There are some specific lines of employment that women have often questioned me about, which I will go on to discuss in more detail. For the effect of work on the pregnant woman in the different trimesters, read Chapters 2 to 4 (pages 85–242). There is one aspect of women and work which I will bring up briefly here: the potential hazards of toxicity in the workplace. If you fear that your place of employment might expose you unnecessarily or dangerously to any toxic chemicals, you should discuss these fears with your obstetrician, employer, or union representative. You can also refer to a government paper on the subject. Called *Guidelines on Pregnancy and Work*, it was published in 1977 by the National Institute for Occupational Safety and Health and the American College of Obstetricians and Gynecologists. (Copies may be obtained from the U.S. Department of Health, Education and Welfare, Center for Disease Control, 5600 Fishers Lane, Rockville, Maryland 20857. Publication no. 78-118.) This publication might help you evaluate your particular situation.

Some specific occupations that might mean a potentially dangerous environment for a pregnancy include those of nurses who work in operating rooms and who are exposed to anesthetic gases, dental assistants and surgeons who work with radiation and mercury, women who work in factories with vinyl chloride or in industries with high levels of radiation. The chances of infertility, repeated spontaneous miscarriages, stillbirths, or birth defects may be slightly increased if you work in these fields. If you are planning a pregnancy, therefore, and your employment is potentially a hazard to the unborn child, make sure to discuss the problems with your obstetrician before conception so that adequate measures can be taken to safeguard your pregnancy.

If you work with radiation, copying machines, or video-display terminals, can you safely get pregnant?

If you work with industrial sources of radiant energy, it is very unlikely that your fetus will suffer any harm, because the levels of radiation are checked and doubled-checked constantly. Work with lasers, ultraviolet, infrared, or microwave radiation is perhaps the most closely monitored of any. Once pregnant, the official view is that no harm can come to your baby unless *you* have been severely burned by radiation. The current opinion of the U.S. Food and Drug Administration (in their *Survey of Photocopier and Related Products,* 1978), is that women who work with Xerox machines every day should have no fears, as long as they keep the top closed when the machine is copying and do not expose themselves to its light.

I am often asked about video-display terminals by my patients. It is the green light that concerns most women, fearing that it might emit more radiation than, say, a color television. A report on VDTs, titled *Potential Health Hazards of Video Display Terminals* (June 1981), has recently come from NIOSH. The conclusion is that VDTs do not emit radiation at levels that present a hazard to exposed employees. However, there is a significant probability of inadvertent contact with a high-voltage source (flyback transformer), so the high-voltage source should be shielded to prevent such contact. (In case that sounds frightening, the flyback transformer is a common component on all TV sets including VDTs.)

If you work with ionizing radiation, you must wear a film badge to monitor the dose. These badges are usually read quarterly, and you can gain access to their records. If you are planning a pregnancy, I advise you to request a monthly badge reading to be sure that the radiation dose remains safe in the period *before* conception. The recommended acceptable level for the embryo or fetus is 0.5 rem (rad) which is equivalent to 1.5 rem for a pregnant woman because of absorption of radiation by the abdominal wall, which usually reduces the fetal dose to the required level. You should, however, remember to add the amount of radiation from any further diagnostic X rays to the amount of the dose you receive at work, and make sure the total does not exceed the recommended level.

If you are concerned about working with ionizing radiation and are not sure of the exact danger of exposure, suggest to your boss or union representative that you be moved to a different department for the period of your pregnancy. Four pregnant employees of the Bell Telephone Company in Canada won the right to refuse to work on cathode ray tube (CRT) terminals without loss of pay, because they felt the equipment *might* emit radiation. Obviously they did not know for sure there was a danger, but their concern was sufficient to persuade their employer.

Will psychological stress at work affect a pregnancy?

Over the centuries pregnant women have handled stress and tension, if not from the demands of a career in a man's world, then from the problems of poverty, of living with a husband in a difficult and sometimes hostile environment, of handling large families, or of dealing with death, illness, and harsh climates. There is, however, some evidence to show that the stresses surrounding work—fatigue from your job; sudden episodes of frenetic activity; high levels of alertness; an uncaring or hostile attitude toward you in pregnancy; the strain of commuting twice a day on the subway, still having to prepare dinner, and maybe look after other members of the family—can become too much in pregnancy.

If you have any of these problems and you have a history of miscarriages, you should try to take it easier during the next pregnancy. Maybe cut down to a 3- or 4-day week, or work those other days at home. If you are struggling against the odds at work, and you suffer early bleeding, cramping, or a deep

59

level of exhaustion, then I advise you think seriously of leaving the job and finding a more restful life style.

Many women these days run themselves into a corner trying to achieve everything. You owe it to yourself and your future child to slow down. Work on your husband to help out more at home. Can you afford to drive to work or take taxis, rather than go by subway? Maybe you should hire help in the home for the duration of the pregnancy, so you do not find yourself cooking and cleaning as well as working all day. An extra expense now may be worth it in the long run. Fatigue and depression in themselves are not going to harm your baby, but they could help lead to a miscarriage, stillbirth, or a low-birthweight baby.

THE HOME AND THE ENVIRONMENT

What potential hazards in the home should be avoided?

The manufacturers of aerosols would probably disagree, but I advise you to limit your use of these sprays in the home before conception and during pregnancy. There are alternatives to most aerosols on the market today, whether they be deodorants, hair sprays, room deodorizers, spray polishes, or oven cleaners. Aerosols now operate on halogenated hydrocarbons (as an alternative to the fluorocarbons that were seen to cause a threat to this planet's ozone layer). This new chemical component creates the propellant and has *not* been implicated in causing any harm to fetus or mother.

However, my feeling is that we are all exposed to invisible sources of potentially harmful chemicals and levels of radiation, and, while pregnant it is advisable to take every possible precaution. Even with all the tests available and even with extra care, some babies are still born with unforeseen and inexplicable rare disorders for which we know no culprit. Some of us in the medical profession believe these new disorders might be due to environmental hazards, which is why I offer these words of warning.

Does that mean *no* aerosols throughout pregnancy? You can use them with caution and sparingly. Remember that during pregnancy you have an increased blood supply and take in more oxygen (this is known as hyperventilating), which could mean you absorb more foreign particles from the air you breathe. So, when you use an aerosol, make sure the room is adequately ventilated, that you inhale as little of the spray as possible, and that you never spray in a closed room or one that has no windows. If you need to use pesticides, ask your husband or someone else to do the spraying and make sure to leave the room or area of the garden being sprayed.

Most couples wish to paint at least the baby's room during pregnancy. You should try to avoid any paint containing lead during pregnancy so as not to be exposed to an excessive level of lead. If you plan to strip off old paint that might contain lead, again I would advise you leave the task to your husband or to professional painters, while you retire.

The stresses and strains of moving house or apartment are best avoided once you are pregnant, but many couples find they have to move during a pregnancy and it is certainly not the end of the world to do so. I have met many women who have gone to live in different countries at various stages of a pregnancy who have experienced no problems. The change of life heralded by the expected baby seems to bring out a sense of adventure and flexibility. As with anything else, of course, there is a word of caution. If you can avoid lifting and carrying boxes of heavy books or kitchen equipment, please do. This is not one of those times to prove you are a liberated woman; leave the heavy work to the movers.

Will you have to give up using a microwave oven once pregnant?

Microwave ovens are a source of radiation, and the FDA has established emission standards for any microwave oven currently on the market. The permissible limits are 5 milliwatts of radiation per square centimeter, measured at 2 inches from the oven surface. Both the authorities and manufacturers believe microwave ovens are safe for home use by humans, whether pregnant or not. However, I believe you should bear in mind that the small amount of radiation emitted by these ovens, together with other invisible sources of radiation (such as that from smoke detectors, for example) *might* add up to a potential hazard for your baby. As I mentioned previously, every now and again babies are born with inexplicable syndromes. My advice, therefore, is to limit the use of your microwave oven to special occasions. Or, if you wish to use the oven on a daily basis, suggest that your husband or other family member operate it on your behalf. The FDA advises that pregnant women should avoid leaning against a microwave oven while it is on and that they avoid standing in front of one for long periods.

Will you have to give up household pets once you are pregnant?

Some animals can transmit diseases that can have a harmful effect on your baby. The most commonly known of these diseases is toxoplasmosis, a parasitic infection that can damage a newborn baby, cause premature labor, or cause stillbirth. It occurs very rarely; the incidence being about 1 in 8,000 in America today, and it is a far less serious condition than is often suggested. Basically, you do not have to get rid of your pets before you get pregnant. Most people are already immune to toxoplasmosis anyway, having lived among household pets as children.

Toxoplasmosis is contracted by ingesting uncooked or badly cooked meats or by exposure to cat feces. (Other household pets such as dogs, goldfish, birds or snakes cannot transmit this infection to humans.) If you have just gotten a cat, or have eaten any steak tartare or raw fish recently and are thinking of trying to get pregnant, you can go for a screening test right now. It is only a question of a blood test (from your arm) which will be sent to a laboratory for analysis. If you already have a cat and are planning a pregnancy, you should avoid emptying the litter tray or handling the feces yourself. And don't eat any uncooked meat or fish.

The only way to find out if you are at risk of getting toxoplasmosis is to be screened for previous exposure, to see if you have the antibodies, either before you get pregnant, or when you first book in with your doctor in pregnancy. For example, here at Mount Sinai we do antibody tests on all mothers-to-be, just to reassure them and to rule out the possibility. Since there is no treatment for toxoplasmosis in pregnancy, if it is found that you do not have the antibodies, then your pregnancy will be watched over more carefully. The degree of the infection that can cause any harm to a baby is very hard to judge, and you may need to see a doctor who is particularly skilled in this area. If you are found to have a very high level of antibodies to toxoplasmosis in pregnancy, a special test for Igm antibodies is done to see if the infection has been recent. If so, termination may have to be discussed.

Is it safe to swim while pregnant?

Sometimes the questions I am asked stem from old wives' tales. If you do go swimming—and swimming is one of the best forms of exercise for the pregnant woman—water will not enter the vagina, nor will it get into the bloodstream through the extra veins in that area of your body. Swimming is quite safe.

May you use saunas, hot tubs, or whirlpools while pregnant?

Among the health-conscious, saunas, hot tubs, and whirlpool baths are very popular. Although I cannot say with one hundred percent accuracy that they are harmful to your pregnancy, I must emphasize that they have been implicated in fetal abnormalities, particularly those of the baby's nervous system.

When your body is subjected to extreme heat over a lengthy period, you may become dangerously overheated, (a condition known as hyperthermia); the same condition may affect the fetus. I therefore advise against using any of the above devices while you are pregnant. If you are accustomed to taking saunas and feel you would really miss them during pregnancy, then do not stay in for more than ten minutes altogether.

May you use Sunray lamps?

Although Sunray lamps are becoming increasingly popular as paler-skinned people attempt to keep that "healthy" tan all year round, the FDA has made quite a strong statement urging caution in their use. Sunray lamps have a strong association with the increasing rates of skin cancer affecting this country, for they expose the body to unusually high levels of ultraviolet radiation. Ultraviolet is a different form of radiation from the infrared used in X rays and has not been specifically associated with birth defects. However, my advice would be not to use Sunray lamps during a pregnancy, as there are dangers of overheating your body temperature, and we have no idea of the long-term culmulative effect of the potentially carcinogenic rays on either you or the fetus.

Can you have a permanent or dye your hair?

Permanents are perfectly safe in pregnancy, but if you have any fears about their long-term effects, let me advise you to wait till after the first 3 months are over, and the period of organogenesis has passed.

Hair dyes are more controversial. The FDA has been urging that a health warning be printed on the packages of commercially available hair dyes that contain coal tar, advising consumers that these dyes may be dangerous to their health. The fear is that such hair dyes are carcinogens. But the cosmetics industry has successfully fought the FDA, and these dyes have not been removed from the market, nor has the warning been printed on the packaging. If you use hair dyes regularly, I suggest that you read the contents on the package carefully for the duration of the pregnancy, and that you do not use coal-tar-based dyes during this period.

Can you watch TV safely for long periods?

Television rays, even from color television, have not been shown to be a form of ionizing radiation. It is not harmful to sit within several feet of a screen, even for long periods. The only danger is to your back, as the familiar pose of watching TV slumped on a sofa is decidedly bad for the lower back, particularly if you are pregnant. If TV is your addiction, may I suggest you sit on the floor, with your back against the sofa; or that you sit on a firm chair with your feet on a low stool. You need to keep your back firm and your legs slightly raised to help circulation and to ease strain on the lower back.

What problems will women who already have small children encounter?

Second-time mothers have a much harder time than first-timers, particularly if their first child is still a toddler. They are likely to feel much more tired, and potentially could suffer more back pain. My only advice is that you pay extra care to your back and to how you lift your child. When the situation requires it, always bend down on your heels and scoop the child up, so you raise both the child and yourself from the squatting position. It may seem harder that way, but it will protect your back from too much strain, as you take the weight on the knees and not on the lower back. If you bend over from the waist and lift the child from mid-height, you will be putting too much strain on your back muscles while they no longer have the help of sturdy stomach muscles. The real favor you can do yourself in a second pregnancy is not to encourage back pain, which may be a problem in labor or postpartum if you are not careful now.

What about environmental hazards?

If there were a chance of moving to a healthier environment I am sure you would jump at it. But we all know that housing, financial problems, and jobs often rule out any such choice. Most of us are exposed to the fumes from thousands of automobiles and trucks thundering through our environments every day. Most of us live by or near enough to some major manufacturing or nuclear plant to be affected in different ways.

If you are unfortunate enough to believe you have been or are being, exposed to either dangerous levels of toxic chemicals in your environment or to nuclear radiation; if you are struggling with inexplicable infertility; if you have had a previous child with a birth defect; or if you have had three or more spontaneous miscarriages, I advise you to see your doctor and discuss it openly with him or her. Maybe your infertility or miscarriage problem is not linked with any environmental factor and can be treated medically.

Where there is concern as to the unborn baby's health because of some environmental exposure, the pregnancy should be managed by the doctor as a high-risk pregnancy, with investigations by ultrasound and amniocentesis.

In the Beginning . . .

GENETICS COUNSELING

Genetics counseling before pregnancy is still a new science, but it is an increasingly sophisticated and valuable part of modern obstetric care. Unless you fall into the group of older first-time mothers (thirty-five or over), the chances of your being referred to the genetics department of a major hospital are quite slight. But if your doctor does suggest it, for any of the reasons you will read about later in this section, I do hope you will not be unduly concerned or worry that something must definitely be wrong with either you or your husband (or your future baby). Genetics counseling is used mainly as a screening test to discover beforehand whether there is, or is likely to be, a problem. There is no stigma attached to the process, and no reason to be apprehensive. If you read further on in this section, I believe you will find the prospect of the counseling reassuring and encouraging rather than cause for concern.

What is genetics counseling?

To some people the term *genetics counseling* may have an aura of the forbidden or unethical—like that of the controversial issue of genetic engineering. But please be reassured: this type of counseling has nothing to do with trying to breed a master race, or dabbling with genetics in any serious form. It is a way of reading the body's signals so that you can prevent a tragedy that *need not happen* in your family.

At a counseling session, you will be interviewed about your own and your husband's family histories. From that information the counselor will assess whether there are any indications that you might be at risk of having a child with some inborn disorder. If so, blood tests will be taken from your arm (and perhaps your husband's). The blood will be analyzed in a special laboratory, and you will be notified of the results within a few weeks.

But let me begin by explaining the area of knowledge that enables your counselor to evaluate you both as prospective parents. Genetics can be a difficult subject to grasp, but bear with it. It becomes fascinating with understanding.

Our bodies are constructed of millions of cells, living, dying, changing all the time. Some cells live for a few months, others for years—like the egg cells which can live for up to 45 or 50 years in the human female. All our body cells contain chromosomes, long threadlike structures that operate in pairs and look something like two arms. The genes—containing the DNA code that imprints physical characteristics; the color of our hair, and eyes, our blood type, etc.; and, to an arguable degree, the form of our personality—are attached to the chromosomes in hundreds of small dots that are much too minuscule to be seen by the human eye.

Unlike the genes, the chromosomes are distinguishable under a microscope. As far back as the 1880s, it was discovered that these threadlike structures will absorb a special kind of dye and become visible. (The derivation of the name is from the Greek *chroma*, meaning color, and *soma*, meaning body.) Today more sophisticated techniques have been evolved but the chromosomes are still basically stained and investigated under magnification. A researcher can detect whether any individual chromosomes are damaged, and whether the pairs make up the right order and number.

In the human body there are 46 chromosomes per cell. Taking your own body as an example, 23 of your chromosomes were inherited from your mother and 23 from your father, including 1 sex chromosome from each parent. If you inherited 1 X and 1 Y, you became a male; 2 Xs and you became a female.

Each individual human being has 22 sets of pairs known as autosomes, plus its 2 sex chromosomes, which adds up to the total of 46 chromosomes. When we reproduce, our egg and sperm cells cleverly only have one-half of the total, carrying 23 chromosomes (22 half autosomes plus 1 sex chromosome). When the egg and sperm cells join, they lock sides and the 2 sets of 23 create yet another complete individual with 46 chromosomes, including its sexual identity. This process of cell division is called meiosis.

Genetically, therefore, our identity and form come in equal shares from both parents. Random selection decides which 2 cells, with particular genes attached to the chromosomes, meet and mate; that is why we are all so uniquely different. In the struggle to create a new life, moreover, a battle for power takes place between the two sets of inherited genes. As the genes of two individuals combine, those of one must take precedence over those of the other. Certain genes are dominant and others are recessive, for which you could read passive. Recessive genes will lie dormant, sometimes for centuries, having no effect on the way a person looks or behaves. But let fate bring two similar recessive genes together, and all sorts of oddities arise: this is when dark-haired couples give birth to a redhead—and also, unfortunately, when couples who had no idea it could happen to them give birth to a child with some congenital defect.

If there has been no history of birth disorders in either of your families; if you are not among certain ethnic groups; if you have not miscarried more than three times; then the chances of your having a child with a birth disorder are quite remote. But these things do happen. I was very upset when a young couple, both normal middle-class people, happy with their one charming little daughter and eagerly looking forward to their second baby, came to me for that birth.

The mother was in her late twenties, very healthy, and concerned to have the most natural childbirth possible. She performed with great strength throughout the labor and was elated at the easy birth. However, something was wrong with the baby and, with the relevant tests over the next few weeks, it was discovered that the child had a congenital case, albeit a mild

Culture; amniotic fluid

Cells counted 20

Modal no. 46

Karotypes revealed a normal appearing 46,XY, male chromosome complement.

No apparent chromosomal abnormality or re-arrangement was evident in this study.

FIG A

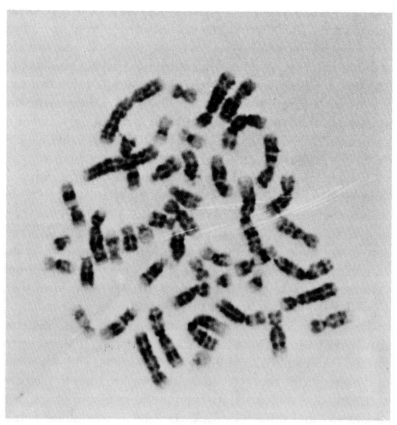

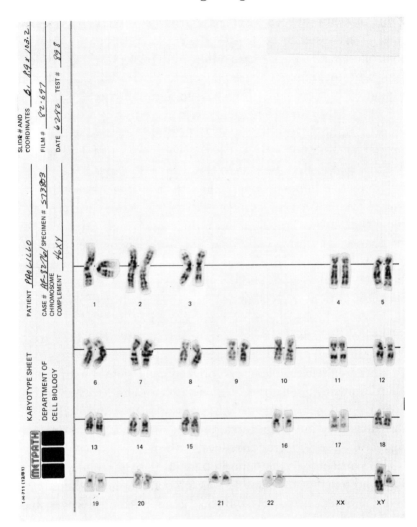

SLIDE # AND COORDINATES 6. 29 x 103.2
FILM # 82-697 TEST # 898
DATE 6292

PATIENT PROLILLO
CASE # AK-82-762 / SPECIMEN # 57383
CHROMOSOME COMPLEMENT 46XY

KARYOTYPE SHEET
DEPARTMENT OF CELL BIOLOGY

METPATH
1-H-711 (12/81)

Fɪɢ B.

The results of your chromosomal analysis will appear in this kind of print-out. Fig. A. shows the cluster of chromosomes in a cell. Fig. B. shows the alignment of autosomes (pairs) made by the geneticist— and all is normal. This baby is a boy as you can see by the X and Y chromosomes in the bottom right hand corner.

form, of cystic fibrosis. The prognosis for their baby is quite good. What used to be a fatal disease in children can now be controlled with special care, diet, and protection from infection. But the parents were obviously distressed that "it had happened to them" and desperate to find out *why*.

Each partner must have carried a recessive gene for cystic fibrosis, through the history of both their families, which had never become apparent as it had always been matched with a dominant gene that overshadowed it. We all carry some recessive defective genes in our bodies. In fact it is estimated that one in twenty Americans today has the cystic fibrosis recessive gene; that means up to 9 to 12 million people are carriers. Yet the chances of mating with a partner also carrying the recessive gene are very low—about 1 in 400. Perhaps, even in their families, other conceptions with the recessive gene had taken place, but they had naturally aborted. Many early miscarriages are of defective embryos that cannot withstand human life.

The couple asked me what their chances were if they tried for another baby. Well, these same people in fact have a 1 in 4 chance—in each pregnancy—of producing a child with 2 normal (dominant) genes; a 2 in 4 chance of a child with 1 recessive and 1 dominant gene, which means the child will be as normal as they are but a carrier; and a 1 in 4 chance of producing a child also suffering from cystic fibrosis.

This particular couple found no joy in the counselor's predictions and felt that the gamble was too dangerous for them ever to risk another pregnancy. But their genetics counselor was able to advise them that if they wished a future pregnancy, it could be undertaken with the assistance of the following evaluation. The pregnancy would be tested in the fourth month (sixteenth week), by amniocentesis. Three or four weeks later, if the fetus was found to have the cystic fibrosis disorder, they would be able to decide at that point whether to take the pregnancy to term or to opt for a therapeutic abortion. The accuracy of this test is still being evaluated.

Cystic fibrosis tends to affect Caucasians. Other common genetic disorders are Tay-Sachs disease, which affects mostly Ashkenzaic Jews of Central and Eastern European origin; sickle-cell anemia, affecting American blacks from Africa, beta-thalassemia, or Cooley's anemia, affecting Italian and Greek Americans of Mediterranean extraction.

All these genetic disorders are on their way to disappearing, as more and more are being detected *before pregnancy,* through widespread screening of informed couples either when they marry or at least prior to trying for a pregnancy.

Some genetic disorders result less directly from the interaction of inherited genes than from a mixture of genetic and environmental factors. I am referring to disorders such as cleft lip or palate, clubfoot, congenital dislocation of the hip, spina bifida (a spinal defect), hydrocephalus (fluid accumulation in the brain) with spina bifida, and an obstruction in the stomach from the small intestine known as pyloric stenosis. These are harder to predict in advance, so if there has been any history of such disorders in either family it is advisable to seek genetic help before conception.

Most parents already into their thirties are very aware of the other most common birth defect, and are anxious to avoid it. Down's syndrome (Mongolism) is not caused by a defective recessive gene, but by chromosomal malformation. The cause can be quite simple, but the effect is devastating.

As I explained earlier, the individual is made up of 46 chromosomes: the 22 pairs of autosomes and 2 single sex chromosomes. Sometimes, during conception, when the bonding of the two sets of 23 chromosomes is taking place, one of the mother's chromosomes may become lodged on the back of another, so that she has a "double" chromosome in the cell. When the sperm's 23 chromosomes enter the picture, the fetus ends up with a cellular structure of 47, not 46, chromosomes. The unfortunate offspring has 3 of what researchers have identified as the Number 21 chromosome—the disorder is also often called "trisomy 21." In the live-born fetus, Mongolism is the result, with its characteristic manifestations of a skin fold at the inner corner of the eyes, a large protruding tongue, and small hands with stubby fingers; most likely there will also be some functional defects of the heart, eyes, and ears, and varying degrees of mental retardation from brain maldevelopment.

Why this happens no one yet knows. Theories include the weakness of an "overripe" egg, meaning one that was fertilized late in the Fallopian tube—by the sperm reaching it on its very last day of its stay in the tubes. As the condition occurs more often in the children of older mothers, it may be due to the ovum having waited four decades in the ovary, and beginning to deteriorate. We do not yet know if the egg cells begin to deteriorate after a certain time. (One well-known doctor has the theory that older mothers, and hence fathers, have intercourse less frequently—so the chances are less that the egg will be fertilized as soon as it leaves the ovary.) I do not support that idea myself! It could also be that some environmental factor affects the ovum at the point of leaving the ovary. Research is investigating the causes of Mongolism right now.

A tendency for Down's syndrome cannot always be discovered *before* a pregnancy. In certain very rare cases the mother has been found to be a carrier of the defective chromosome I described, balanced by a nondefective one. For a parent with such a "balanced translocation," the chances in each conception are 1 in 3 of having a Down's syndrome child; 1 in 3 of having a child who will similarly be a carrier; and 1 in 3 of a perfectly normal child, neither carrier nor affected. In the extremely rare cases of both parents having "balanced translocation," all conceptions will have Down's syndrome. Indeed, there is one reported case of such parents who had five Mongoloid children.

If either of your families has a history of children born brain damaged, with mental retardation, or with such defects as deafness, eye problems, even dwarfism, a genetics counselor will be able to reassure you that all such disorders are *not* transmitted genetically. Your chances of having a healthy normal baby are most likely the same as anyone else's.

Genetics screening: Why are you being advised to attend?

By attending genetics counseling before even trying to get pregnant a couple can reassure themselves about some potential problems and dangers. Do not be afraid that you may be counseled *against* ever having a baby. The counseling acts much more as a preventive measure to show you how it will be *possible*, even though you fall into a high-risk group. Should yours be a high-risk pregnancy, it will be supported and investigated by ultrasound and amniocentesis at every necessary stage. If, in the rare case, it is found at 20 weeks that the growing fetus does have a serious abnormality, you will be offered the choice of therapeutic abortion rather than facing the emotional, physical, and financial burden of bringing such a child into the world.

Certain people are strongly encouraged to attend genetic screening before pregnancy. In particular, I advise screening for couples of ethnic backgrounds related to known genetic diseases. For example, all Jewish couples, or couples where one partner is not Jewish, are advised to be tested for Tay-Sachs disease. Tay-Sachs is an extremely traumatic genetic disorder of progressive cerebral degeneration. The babies are born seemingly normal, but a pediatrician can detect the disorder by checking for a cherry-red spot at the back of the baby's eye. The disease usually manifests itself at about 6 months, when the baby begins to deteriorate; few survive their third or fourth year. Parents who conceive a child with the Tay-Sachs disorder may be totally unaware that they are both carriers, as each has one dominant and one recessive gene—leaving them normal. But when the two Tay-Sachs recessive genes combine, the disease is inevitable. As with cystic fibrosis, the chances of its happening are 1 in 4 with *each* pregnancy.

The incidence of Tay-Sachs carriers among Ashkenazic Jews

is 1 in 30. (Among non-Jews the indence is 1 in 300, which is why the partners in a marriage between Jew and non-Jew should still be investigated.) Many Jewish couples already receive the screening test along with their VD test for a marriage license.

The extensive Tay-Sachs screening program in the U.S. and Canada is bringing about some exciting results. Since 1969, some 200,000 people in the Jewish community have submitted to screening. I have seen just one case of Tay-Sachs in my whole working life, and the disorder is already on the decline because of this effective program. From these screenings, more than 200 couples (who had never had a child) were positively identified as Tay-Sachs carriers. As these carriers have a 1 in 4 chance of having a child with the disorder, these 200 couples were therefore considered to be at high risk. So far we have the figures that of those couples, 600 pregnancies have been tested with amniocentesis and 150 Tay-Sachs births have been prevented. The other 450 pregnancies, however, were known to be normal and indeed the babies were born healthy and without the disorder.

Without the screening programs I doubt those parents who are carriers would dare to have had a baby, let alone more than one. After one child born with Tay-Sachs, it is very hard to take the gamble on risking another pregnancy. The new exciting science of genetic evaluation, with amniocentesis as support, is now enabling couples who would have feared pregnancy before, to have healthy normal children.

Some parents are religiously or philosophically opposed to therapeutic abortion even on such humane grounds. I know that most genetics laboratories ask for a form to be signed agreeing to an abortion if the amniocentesis turns up evidence of Tay-Sachs or other serious disorders. The laboratory and hospitals tend to feel it is not worth the expense and time on their part to make the investigation if it is not to help parents in preventing the enormous overload on emotions, health, and finances caused by the birth of such a child. However, if you are strongly against abortion, even of such a fetus, and yet still wish to be genetically evaluated and tested by amniocentesis, you may ask around the genetics centers at your nearby teaching hospitals to find one sympathetic to your feelings.

There are parents who would still accept the risk of giving birth to a Tay-Sachs baby, but would prefer to have amniocentesis so they may be prepared well in advance for the measures that will have to be taken. I recall one Jewish couple who had already had one normal and one Tay-Sachs child. They knew the risks for their third pregnancy. When we did the biochemical test on the amniotic fluid after amniocentesis, we did indeed find Tay-Sachs again. But they decided not to have the pregnancy aborted and the baby was born with the disorder. They had found a place for the baby in a special home for the incurably ill, where it would spend its 3 years of life. People differ widely on their views over such births and, I do wish to emphasize, no one will force you to abort such a fetus. The choice will always be your own.

Carrier screening before pregnancy is also advised for black people of African descent, as one in ten American black people are carriers of sickle-cell anemia. With this genetic disorder, the individual suffers from a lack of red blood cells. The remaining cells, when short of oxygen, form a sickle or S shape. It is a painful and debilitating disease, though not always fatal, which may appear in infancy but often not till the child is about six years old.

The other ethnic group advised to go for carrier screening are those of Mediterranean extraction, usually Greek or Italian, who may be disposed to the genetic disorder called beta-thalassemia, or Cooley's anemia. With the prospect of the same positive advantages I outlined for Tay-Sachs screening, these groups of parents are made fully aware of the risks and the support system available.

A woman who has had three or more consecutive miscarriages is also advised to go for genetics counseling before trying

WILL MY BABY BE NORMAL?

another pregnancy, particularly if her doctor has found no obvious cause. One of the commonest causes of a first miscarriage is an abnormal chromosomal makeup of the fetus. What might have happened is that, at the birth of one or both of this couple, their chromosomes fell into a wrong arrangement. When they try to have a child, the balance of their combined chromosomes is incompatible with human life and so the product of conception naturally and spontaneously aborts.

If such a chromosomal disorder is discovered, your doctor will know that any future pregnancy must be treated with the utmost care and attention. If a pregnancy should survive till the fourth month, then your physician may investigate the condition of the fetus by amniocentesis to see if the baby you are carrying is healthy and fine. If major chromosomal damage is inescapable, your doctor can advise you in numerous ways and perhaps you will want to consider artificial insemination by donor, or adoption.

On an encouraging note, I just recently delivered a woman of a healthy normal baby who had had seven previous miscarriages. She had had numerous tests and also attended genetics counseling, the result of which was normal. Knowing, therefore, that we were not dealing with some impossible situation, we overcame her negative attitude and she became confident that her pregnancy would be normal. We followed our positive reasoning, recommended periods of prolonged bed rest, tested her regularly with ultrasound, and all went well. This story illustrates that investigations can mean as much when they are negative as when they are positive, and that reassurance is very important.

If you are over thirty-five or your husband is fifty-five or over, you should also consider genetics counseling before a pregnancy, to test for the chances of your conceiving a Down's syndrome (Mongoloid) child. Perhaps it seems strange to you to think of a couple, trying for the first time to have a baby at what we call "advanced" maternal (or paternal) age, seeking such counseling before even trying to conceive—most people in that situation will be concerned first with infertility, not with abnormality. But the age of both parents does play a significant role in the well-being of the fetus (see page 162).

A woman of thirty-seven with her new husband of forty-five came to see me a while ago to discuss whatever problems they might encounter in a pregnancy. I advised them to seek genetics counseling just to reassure themselves. Even at this woman's age, the risk of having a Down's syndrome child is not high (see table on page 165).

Recently, the mother of a twelve-year-old boy gave a great boost to anxious "older" mothers. Her son was on TV as the youngest child *ever* to enroll at New York University. At twelve, he has an IQ of something over 190—genius level. The mother, who had already had four children before conceiving him, had prepared herself to have problems with this fifth child. She was forty, and there was history of mental retardation on both sides of the family. She fully expected that this "late" baby might be mentally retarded. However, when he was six months old she realized she had quite a different problem on her hands: an extremely gifted child.

There is certainly nothing *wrong* with having a baby at forty or even forty-five. In my work in New York and in London, I have met journalists, editors, doctors, nurses, public-relations people, musicians, ballerinas, and yes, even housewives, who have given birth to their first or their fifth child at age forty or more. The message is that it can be done—just be aware of the precautions and the support that is available.

Couples who are closely related—such as first cousins, second cousins, uncle and niece—should also consider genetics counseling. First cousins have one eighth of their genes in common. We all have several defective recessive genes buried in our cells, which can only cause a disorder if one of these becomes part of a recessive pair. But first cousins, with so many of their genes in common, run a much greater risk of this occurrence. A man with a recessive gene for cystic fibrosis, for example, who has only a 1 in 400 chance of marrying a carrier with a similar gene when he marries an unrelated woman, shoots those odds to 1 in 8 when he marries a first cousin. The risk of chromosomal abnormalities in the offspring of the same couple is similarly greatly increased—from 1 in 1,600 to 1 in 32, for each pregnancy.

Of course, if you have already given birth to an abnormal child of any kind, even if it was in a previous marriage, do go now for genetics counseling to assess the risk, so that you can make an informed decision about whether you should attempt another pregnancy. If someone else in your family has been born with a disorder or given birth to a child with a disorder, you might consider early counseling too. Carrier genes very seldom affect cousins, aunts, uncles. But if you would like to be reassured, why not seek advice before you become pregnant?

What will happen at genetics counseling?

You will sit down around a table and be asked questions about your family pedigrees. The counselor will fill out a detailed report on both your family histories, as far back as is possible— preferably up to three generations. The counselor will need to know general medical details about any branch of either family; about the number of miscarriages, stillbirths, and children who died in infancy; about the general health of your parents, brothers, and sisters. You can obtain free forms called Family Medical Records from the March of Dimes so that you can begin working on those histories now.

If the counselor feels there is any need to investigate you further before you become pregnant, a blood test will be taken, sent to a laboratory, and examined for many different metabolic and chromosomal disorders. At present the results from that blood test will take a few days.

Why does it take so long? From your blood the genetics technicians take the white blood cells, which are then grown in the laboratory, rather as you might grow plants from seeds. Over a period of weeks the cells begin to divide and make more cells. At that point the cells are crushed, spread out, and, through a microscope, the distinct pattern of the chromosomes is identified. They are matched in pairs, visually. The technicians are looking for any abnormality in the arrangement of the 22 pairs of autosomes and the 2 single sex chromosomes (see picture, pages 70–71).

Why is it more valuable to do this before a pregnancy than during one? A Jewish couple presenting themselves at a genetics center for Tay-Sachs screening, before conceiving, will be tested by a blood sample from the arm, as described above. The man is tested first, and, if he is found to be a carrier then his wife is tested. The geneticist will be looking for an enzyme which, if missing, indicates that the subject is a Tay-Sachs carrier. It is a simple test, causing no pain (other than that of the needle in the arm) and the results will be available in a couple of days. However, if the wife is already pregnant when her husband proves to be a Tay-Sachs carrier, her blood test is no longer reliable as the presence of pregnancy hormones may alter the results. For the pregnant woman, therefore, the only testing done for Tay-Sachs is amniocentesis, and that will not be before the sixteenth week of pregnancy. However, new work suggests that the blood test on women may be satisfactory even when they are pregnant.

Amniocentesis is now used quite commonly (see section on amniocentesis, page 161) to investigate pregnancies that show any indication of a possible disorder. But the problem with having to wait for the results of amniocentesis is one of time.

Once you are pregnant, the geneticist will be working with fetal cells that have been washed off the baby's body surface.

They are found in the amniotic fluid in which the fetus lives and which has been drawn from the mother's uterus. Amniocentesis is a very safe procedure for both mother and baby. The only problem, as I said, is one of time; and this can be compounded if anything goes slightly wrong. From the time the cells are taken in the amniotic fluid, it takes at least 3 to 4 weeks to get a positive analysis, which is a long time in the course of a pregnancy. It is a particularly long time if the pregnancy has to be aborted when a serious defect has been discovered. To overcome this lengthy wait, doctors right now are considering other techniques including the use of biopsies, which means taking a piece of tissue directly from the fetal body surface, or from placental vessels inside the uterus. This procedure, known as fetoscopy, will be explained more fully later in our discussion of the birth process (see page 189). Its virtue is that the results come through much more quickly—within a week. Since fetoscopy is at the experimental stage, do not expect your doctor to conduct a routine fetal biopsy in the second trimester for a few years yet.

For now, amniocentesis itself is an exciting enough development; one that eases the burden on the parents of waiting and worrying till the end of the pregnancy. But I must also explain why the length of time can be a nuisance, so that you fully understand we cannot guarantee miracles with the procedure. The problems arise if the amniocentesis does not work. There are times when the culture of the chromosomes performed after the amniotic fluid has been drawn does not take. Some of the mother's cells may grow instead of the baby's. There may not be enough cells in the sample of fluid for adequate analysis. Or the mere growing of the cells outside the body may cause its own aberrations. For any of these reasons, the amniocentesis would have to be repeated and another 3 or 4 weeks will pass before you would know the results. It is really very sad when this happens, for your pregnancy would have reached at least 23 weeks and, if the results then showed a birth disorder, or chromosomal damage to your baby, you or your doctor may consider it too late for a therapeutic abortion. There would then be no choice but to wait for the birth.

But the success rate of cultures taken in amniocentesis is remarkably high, so do not worry. Generally speaking, it is more than 98 percent successful with a single sample of at least 10 milliliters of amniotic fluid (30 milliliters of fluid is usually withdrawn). If the fluid is absolutely clear then the success rate is nearer 100 percent. However, there are those rare occasions when tissue cultures do not succeed.

How do you find a genetics center?

If you live outside of a major urban area and far from a large teaching hospital, first ask your doctor if he or she knows of the nearest genetics center. You can also contact the March of Dimes for their International Directory of Genetic Services. Not all laboratories have the ability to do every test. The March of Dimes list will show which ones routinely do the thirty different enzyme assays for inborn metabolic errors. It is preferable that the center be attached to a teaching hospital, as geneticists at these centers have access to diagnostic expertise in pediatrics, neurology, ophthalmology, cardiology, and any number of other disciplines. As extensive research is ongoing in these teaching hospitals, into the etiology and epidemiology of birth defects, bear in mind more and more information is becoming available to the geneticist.

New genetics centers are opening up nationwide and more geneticists are being trained to meet the increasing need. Most centers began only being able to do a few culture analyses a week, and they imposed strict limits on *who* would be tested. But with improved facilities, and in the face of the growing demand, they are now relaxing those limits.

What will it cost you? The costs will no doubt vary among different centers, but the approximate prices in New York City at time of writing are as follows: genetic studies of amniotic fluid cells—$500 (includes genetics counseling, chromosome studies, alpha-fetoprotein, and other tests). Chromosome studies on adults, extra to that of the fetal cells, usually cost about $175 for each parent studied. Chromosome analysis alone, before a pregnancy: $150 each ($300 a couple). If genetics counseling is necessary before a pregnancy, an additional $75. The fee for Tay-Sachs screening before a pregnancy is about $40 per person. The physician's fee for performing an amniocentesis is around $100. You will have to check with your insurance company for the extent of your coverage.

CHAPTER

2

The First Trimester

1–12 WEEKS

The reproductive miracle is about to take place. Some of the symptoms of pregnancy will bring with them discomfort and irritation at your inability to perform as usual, but they usually bring fascination as well. The medical story that is beginning to unfold is becoming less and less a mystery to doctors as we learn more and more about the physiological changes going on in your body; but all this new knowledge makes the process no less remarkable. The changes set in motion by pregnancy differ from any others in life. Dramatic as they are, they are also temporary. Your body will return to normal after the birth. Throughout the pregnancy you will be building up reserve stores of certain nutrients to cover your baby's potential needs.

The fetus is not, as has commonly been held, a parasite, but a being capable of creating and controlling its own environment; and that environment is *you*! And you thought it was a helpless little scrap of tissue and blood!

Physiological changes in the mother

Mood changes: You may become slightly irritable, or very drowsy, conditions that can be aggravated by the nausea or vomiting of early pregnancy. And your libido may decrease. We used to ascribe these reactions to psychological pressures, but now it is thought that the physiology of the brain goes through major metabolic changes with each stage of pregnancy (compare the joy and fulfilled feeling of the second trimester to the urgent desire for it all to be over of the third).

Breasts: Owing to changes in the circulating hormones, such as estrogen and progesterone, the breasts become enlarged. They take in an increase of fatty deposits and of tissue for the milk ducts. The areola, the area surrounding the nipple, becomes darker and develops little nodules called Montgomery's tubercles. After 6 weeks of pregnancy, a softer, lighter area known as the secondary areola develops around the darker skin. Usually there is not any fluid secretion from the nipples until the second trimester.

Pigmentation: On light-skinned women, a slightly darker coloration can appear on the nose, forehead, and upper lip, in a butterfly configuration. This is called chloasma and usually fades after pregnancy. Pigmentation also may deepen on the line of skin from the umbilicus to the vulva (your navel to your pubic hair), or sometimes even higher up the belly. This *linea nigra* is obviously more noticeable the fairer the person. It should fade after pregnancy, though in many women the nipples and *linea nigra* may remain particularly pigmented. Most moles (or beauty spots) will also darken, owing to a reorganization of melanin in the cells of the skin.

Change of appetite: This condition is known as pica, which means changed or bizarre taste. It has really less to do with the desire for esoteric foods or drinks than with temporary aversions. These days we do not seem to hear so much about women craving strawberries or oysters. But certainly their appetites do change. They may go off coffee which they normally love, or alcohol. Likewise they may desire foods they detest when not pregnant. Some women will eat more and some eat less (these latter women may even lose weight in the first trimester of pregnancy).

Sweat glands: Pregnant women may perspire more than they do in the nonpregnant state. Pregnancy induces a hypermetabolic condition, which means the body accelerates all its functions.

Reproductive tract: The labia may become slightly swollen, and some women may develop varicose veins of the labia (just as you can get varicose veins in the legs). They are nothing to worry about and shrink after pregnancy. If they cause discomfort they can be relieved by rest. The vagina will become very acid during pregnancy as a protection against some infections. However, the acidity also promotes fungal growth, which quite frequently causes a very itchy and uncomfortable discharge. The discharge is easily treated.

Uterus: The uterus, or womb, enlarges even in early pregnancy though it cannot be felt through the abdomen till the end of the first trimester (12 weeks). Your doctor may assess its growth by vaginal examination before the end of the first trimester if it is necessary.

Bladder: One of the first signs of pregnancy is the desire to pass urine more often than is normal. This is known as bladder irritability, which is different from cystitis (a bladder infection), as there will be no burning of urine as it passes. The cause of the irritability is not known. It may be due to hormonal changes or to the increasing amount of fluid passed by the kidneys.

Breathing: When pregnant, your breathing is more rapid, which helps to blow off the carbon dioxide in your body. In turn, this helps the fetus get rid of its acids, and with the improved maternal oxygenation the fetus is assured of a better oxygen supply, too.

Minor discomforts: Many of the minor discomforts of pregnancy are apparent in the first trimester. Some of these have been covered in the sections above. They also include: bleeding gums, nosebleeds, blocked nose (from congestion of the mucous membranes), nausea, vomiting, constipation (from decreased bowel contractions), excess salivation, acid vaginal discharge, and frequent passage of urine. Hemorrhoids may also be a discomfort. Any of these "minor" problems may increase with successive pregnancies, and, if you have a twin pregnancy, they are likely to be more noticeable—after all, everything is doubled.

Changes in the developing baby

The development of the embryo begins from the moment the sperm and egg meet in the outer part of the Fallopian tube following your ovulation in midcycle. The cells that have met, fuse and start dividing, so that after 4 days there is a mass of cells called the blastocyst. This develops little fingers called chorionic villi, which are necessary for the embedding of the developing baby. After 7 days, the embryo reaches the uterus. The villi start burrowing into the lining of the uterus and the egg gets a new source of nutrition by opening into the mother's blood vessels.

You, the mother, will still not have missed a period at this stage of implantation, which is why I have previously emphasized that you must not take any drugs or medication in the latter half of a menstrual cycle in which you could be pregnant.

The mass of cells begins to form into a fetus and an amniotic cavity. As the fetus develops, a cord goes out to the brand-new, not-yet-formed placenta; amniotic fluid is put into production, and the amniotic and chorionic membranes appear.

Second week after conception: (Again, this method of dating should not be confused with traditional pregnancy dating, which is from the first day of your last period. For that method of dating just add 2 weeks to these figures.) The pregnancy has now grown to the extent it can be seen with the naked eye. The ovary contains the tiny cystlike corpus luteum from which the egg was expelled (see page 9), which maintains the early pregnancy and produces progesterone that stops you from menstruating.

Third week after conception: Baby is 2 millimeters long. Its main parts are just starting to take shape: the spine, nervous system, head, and trunk.

Fourth week after conception: The head is formed, the chest, abdomen, brain, and spinal cord are completed. The limb buds begin to appear and, by the end of the week, the heart is formed and circulation has begun to be put in motion.

Fifth week after conception: The limbs have developed. The baby has its own blood cells circulating throughout its body. Its intestines have grown but they are not yet in their proper place. The fetus is now about 1.3 centimeters (about half an inch) long.

Sixth week after conception: The heart beats strongly. All the major internal organs, including the lungs, are formed. Growth of the eyes and ears is now taking place. Its length is 2.2 centimeters (nearly an inch) long. This, by the way, is a very vulnerable time for the developing embryo and the very worst time to get German measles because the eyes and ears are forming. An ultrasound examination will now show the fetal heart pulsing and the viability of a pregnancy can be assessed by such a scan.

Seventh week after conception: By the end of the week, the fetus will be about 3 centimeters long (just over 1¼ inches), and will weigh 2 grams (less than an eighth of an ounce). Although the baby moves now, you will not feel it for some time yet.

Eighth week after conception: The umbilical cord is formed but there is still no placenta. The fetus is 4½ centimeters (1¾ inches) long, and weighs 5 grams (less than a quarter of an ounce).

Ninth week after conception: The fetus is recognizable as a human being. Its eyes are completely formed and it is now classified as a fetus, no longer as an embryo. It will be about as long as your little finger, 5½ centimeters (2¼ inches) and will weigh 10 grams (one third of an ounce). Once the fetus has been around for these 9 weeks, everything is formed, and the period of *organogenesis* (see page 8) is said to be over. From now on, major congenital catastrophes should not be able to form other than those brought about by environmental hazards and prematurity.

Tenth week after conception: The face is completely formed. The external genital organs are growing. The baby is 6½ centimeters (2½ inches) long, and weighs 18 grams (nearly two thirds of an ounce).

Eleventh week after conception: The sex of the baby would now be obvious by ultrasound and it will be about 7½ centimeters (3 inches) long and will weigh 30 grams (about an ounce).

Twelfth week after conception: At this stage, which we call the end of the first trimester, all the fetal organs are formed but the baby is still immature. It cannot live independently outside of the uterus. The uterus is now so enlarged that it begins to protrude out of the pelvis, and your doctor will be able to palpate it abdominally (feel the uterus with his or her hands). The uterus also contains about 100 milliliters (less than quarter of a pint) of amniotic fluid.

From now on, the organs themselves, besides enlarging, develop the baby's capacity for independent life, which helps to ensure its survival.

PREGNANCY TESTS

How will you know you are really pregnant?

Any woman will have her secret moments of conviction that she is pregnant from some time in the middle of the month when she might have conceived, to those tremulous days of awaiting the menstrual period. The whole course of events over the next week or so, as she visits the bathroom with fear and her fingers crossed, praying *not* to see the red stain that will likely mark the end to this waited-for pregnancy, is a very private and anxious time for a woman and not something that can be shared with her doctor or even, in most cases, with her husband. Maybe a close woman friend, or relative, will be let in on the secret—"It still has not come. I must be three or four days overdue by now," as she waits until the point comes when she feels confident enough to express her emotions.

In the meantime, the sensations that will have indicated possible pregnancy will have included a feeling of dizziness or light-headedness that might just last a few minutes or be constant, and a sense of heaviness and overtiredness. Her breasts may seem much harder and more definitely swollen; she may notice veins that are very blue and that stand out like the map of a river all over her chest and breasts. Her nipples may be extremely hard and may tingle. A pregnant woman may experience less of the tense irritability associated with the premenstrual syndrome, and she may find she has an increasing aversion to alcohol, cigarette smoke, and social small talk. Very often a woman really begins to be suspicious if she has just a show of blood around the time of her expected period, but had none of the usual premenstrual symptoms.

The only way to be sure of a pregnancy early on is to have a pregnancy test performed (at absolutely no risk to you or the baby, and at little cost). I doubt I have to persuade any woman today to get such a test done. Most women are extremely anxious to have a pregnancy confirmed in their mind (it seems to take forever to show in the body at this stage), and they want to have the earliest result possible.

A generation ago, the only confirmation of pregnancy was when the woman had missed two or more periods and presented herself at the doctor's office, with an already swelling belly. At which point she was usually told to go away and return 7 or 8 months later for the delivery! These days, the very opposite is true of prenatal care. Your doctor will want you to find out as early as possible, and to come in for your first pregnancy visit. No waiting till you feel nauseated and then decide you had better attend the doctor's office or clinic. Early management of pregnancy is vitally important for a safe and healthy pregnancy, for a fit and normal baby. And good prenatal management is now considered more important than what happens at labor and delivery.

Is there any risk in delaying the diagnosis of pregnancy?

As I have explained, the most important time of fetal development is in the very early few days before you even know you are pregnant. After conception, the fertilized egg takes 6 to 7 days to travel down the Fallopian tube before implanting itself in the uterus. There, it is kept alive by the corpus luteum and the pregnancy is maintained by the new hormones that are immediately put into production: progesterone and human chorionic gonadotrophin (HCG). The fertilized egg develops at its most rapid rate during the first 4 weeks after conception.

During these first four weeks, the nervous system begins to develop: the brain, spinal cord and nerves take shape; the eyes and ears begin to bud; the heart begins to beat; and the buds of arms and legs become visible. If you were to take drugs— either medically prescribed, or socially for pleasure—during this period, you might inadvertently alter the fate of your baby's future without realizing the harm you were causing.

So, my advice is—get the earliest pregnancy test possible. You no longer have to wait till you are the traditional 2 weeks overdue from the first missed period. There is a sophisticated and fast pregnancy test available which is not done on the urine but on the blood. This test is 100 percent accurate and is available through most medical schools and commercial laboratories.

I do appreciate that many women feel insecure at this stage of their lives and would prefer to have a pregnancy test done in secrecy or at least in privacy. There is a great attraction, therefore, to the commercially available "home pregnancy tests." However, these are urine tests which necessitate the traditional delay, and they are easily wasted due to mistiming, or spillage. If you do not want to see your own doctor, or do not yet have a gynecologist, free pregnancy testing services are often available through a students' or women's center in major cities or larger towns.

Let me now explain how the HCG blood test works and why it is 100 percent accurate. There is nothing alarming about this test. It only requires a small blood sample from your arm. You can eat and drink as you wish beforehand. The results are usually available within an hour or so. The cost at present is about ten dollars. You need a doctor's authorization before going to a laboratory for this test.

The test measures the amount of human chorionic gonadotrophin in the blood. HCG is produced by the new pregnancy as soon as it embeds in the lining of the uterus on the twenty-first day of the menstrual cycle. The test, therefore, is possible 7 days after conception or 7 days before you would miss a period. The amount of HCG increases daily and, by the twenty-eighth day, when you would expect your normal menstrual flow, there is a sufficient amount present to suppress your period—which is how you come to "miss" it. By the thirty-fifth day, 1 week after the missed period, HCG can be found in concentrated form in a urine specimen (hence the timing of the urine pregnancy tests). Recent discoveries have shown that, by the method known as radioimmunoassay, concentrations of HCG can be reliably detected even earlier—only 9 days after midcycle, which corresponds to 8 days after conception and 1 day after implantation.

The new blood test, therefore, can give you a positive or negative result some 5 to 6 days *before* you would expect to miss a period.

The reason I so strongly advise finding out sooner rather than later was re-established when a tearful patient in her mid-thirties came to see me. Was she pregnant or not? She was just married and very surprised at the fast turnabout of events in her life, yet thrilled it was all happening. Like many women in their thirties, she had led a peripatetic and sometimes rather traumatic life, which included a history of three abortions, various problems with contraception, and a frequently broken heart. Now things appeared to be going so well, she was finding it difficult to relax in the news of the pregnancy and enjoy it. Anxiety and guilt were flooding to the forefront. She was convinced that either she was not pregnant or that she was doing some harm to the baby.

The cause of the anxiety? Her period was 10 days overdue, her breasts were swollen, and based on the experience of the past three pregnancies, which had been terminated, she did feel pregnant. However, she had invested in a home pregnancy test kit and the result had been negative. Worse, there was a crisis going on at her work. It was a time in which she wanted to look her best. But she was coming down with flu, felt miserable and depressed, and wondered whether she could take aspirin or a flu medication. There was a tone of desperation in her voice.

First, I reassured her that to take some Tylenol or paracetamol, rather than aspirin, for the symptoms of flu, would be the best thing for her. Performing poorly in her work, at this critical stage of her career, would not be beneficial to her or the pregnancy. Second, I told her that if she had come to me earlier we could have diagnosed this pregnancy a week or more ago, dealt with her fears about the flu, and eased her anxiety.

I do appreciate that the period of waiting and wondering can be a lonely and anxiety-making time. In the case of this patient, just to know that a doctor understood seemed to be enough. The outcome of the blood test was a confirmed pregnancy. Suddenly, the heaviness, depression, soreness of breasts, and general uncertainty about her life fell into place. It was the pregnancy, added to the depressing symptoms of flu, that was making her feel this way. In the end, she decided against taking any medication, even though I reassured her that neither the flu nor the medication prescribed would harm the fetus. But she preferred to play it safe, and to struggle through what she now saw as "only flu"!

SOME DIFFICULTIES OF EARLY PREGNANCY

Nausea

What effect does nausea or vomiting have on pregnancy?

Although we do not know quite why they occur, nausea and vomiting have been accepted as a part of normal pregnancy and should not cause you concern except for the personal discomfort. The nausea usually vanishes by the twelfth week, though it can linger on in some until as late as the sixteenth week. It is very rare for mild nausea or vomiting to continue further into the pregnancy, though again this can happen and is not really a cause for concern. The level of nausea experienced can vary with each pregnancy.

Some women feel only mild nauseous sensations, a change

in taste buds (often described as a metallic taste), and they go off certain foods and substances—such as milk, fatty foods, coffee, alcohol, or the smell of cigarette smoke. Some women vomit once a day, in the morning—which is why this disturbance has become known as morning sickness—but nausea can strike any time of day or night. Others vomit three or four times a day, regularly after meals. Although it is obviously unpleasant, the vomiting is not usually as desperate as in the nonpregnant state. Generally, women seem able to keep a sense of humor about their discomfort. Their doctor can only reassure them that it will pass. Though one woman I constantly reassured in this way ended up saying wryly, "Yes, in nine months time!" She vomited regularly throughout her pregnancy.

I must emphasize that mild vomiting at such a scale will not harm your pregnancy, unless it becomes severe or you take some untried and potentially harmful drug to control it. Generally women find they can adjust their diet and life to accommodate the problem. It has been proved beneficial to eat regular small carbohydrate meals, every 2 hours or so. Eating so frequently means that your blood sugar level never drops, and this will ease the discomfort. Try to avoid large rich meals. Do not eat sugary foods, as they disturb the blood sugar level. Avoid those smells or foods that turn you off, whether they are greasy foods, fatty meat, milk, tea, coffee, wine, or just garlic. The nausea may also be accompanied by flatulence, and you may find that certain vegetables, or spicy foods, render you quite incapacitated.

Do not worry about your nutrition too much in these months of pregnancy. The fetus will not be harmed, nor will the pregnancy, if you have to omit certain foods. It is difficult to give good advice on controlling the nausea as there is no hard and fast rule. Each woman's experience is different. Follow your own taste buds. But do try to keep some food in your stomach.

What about antiemetics (medications against nausea and vomiting)? Many American women have taken Bendectin (an antihistamine with Vitamin B-6) to relieve nausea and vomiting in early pregnancy. However, there have been recent press reports that questioned its safety without really proving its danger. As a result, the American College of Obstetricians and Gynecologists declared that there is no harmful fetal effect linked with the use of Bendectin in early pregnancy, but studies continue.

If you really feel in need of a medication, do consult your obstetrician. There will always be some new antivomiting agent on the market, and you must avoid using untried drugs in early pregnancy. If you can come to terms with the discomfort without any interference from a drug, I think you will feel safer and happier about the pregnancy in the long run. If your doctor has prescribed pregnancy supplements (multivitamins) and they make you feel nauseated, you may want to postpone taking them until the nausea ends.

Hyperemesis gravidarum: In some very rare instances, about 3 out of 1,000 pregnant women, vomiting is very severe and intractable, not only after meals but even between meals. Nutrition for these women can be disturbed, which ultimately can lead to a serious condition of dehydration from the loss of body minerals and chemicals. The condition itself is known as hyperemesis gravidarum and its cause is unknown. It is difficult to diagnose since no one knows at exactly what point regular vomiting becomes serious. If you are vomiting more than three or four times daily, your doctor should see you regularly to watch for such symptoms as weight loss, falling blood pressure, loss of skin elasticity, and dry membranes. You should also be checked for any general disease that might be aggravating the vomiting. If you are vomiting at a dangerous level, you will probably be given an ultrasound scan as you could have a rare condition called a "molar" pregnancy, which is a tumor on the placenta; or there may be a multiple pregnancy.

Treatment for hyperemesis gravidarum is very specialized and may require hospitalization. Fluids will be given intravenously to replace and maintain normal body levels. Medication will be given to stop the vomiting. The condition should not alter or increase your chance of miscarrying, or of giving birth to an underweight baby or one with any congenital abnormalities. The main concern is for your health and condition. With our better understanding of the condition, however, hyperemesis has become quite uncommon.

Will an absence of nausea increase your chance of miscarrying?

The most common indication of pregnancy for any woman, whether or not she has a laboratory confirmation already in hand, is the slight change in the taste buds that comes between 10 days to 2 weeks after the first missed period and is followed by the onset of nausea or vomiting.

For those women who have suffered the psychological turn-abouts of negative pregnancy tests becoming positive, and the ensuing doubt that they really are pregnant, the onset of such unpleasant symptoms can be ironically welcome. However, many women suffer *no* such symptoms—in fact, only half of all pregnant women experience any nausea or vomiting. It is very often these women who come to see me in great distress as they have heard from their mothers or best friends that they are quite likely to miscarry if they suffer no nausea at all.

This is still a controversial area of obstetrics, as there is no scientific reason why women should feel nausea or vomit, other than the presence of the pregnancy hormones causing some digestive upsets possibly due to a change in brain metabolism (see page 86). But we doctors have definitely gone beyond the "It's only psychological because you are worried about the pregnancy" attitude. In the past, many doctors presumed that the absence of nausea as a symptom must mean an insufficient level of the pregnancy hormones, and they warned women of the threat of miscarriage. But statistically there is as yet no evidence to link early miscarriage with absence of nausea. Women who suffer no nausea or vomiting at all have perfectly normal pregnancies and perfectly normal babies. Similarly, there is another commonly held theory that if you suffer bleeding in early pregnancy (see pages 99–102) but still feel nauseated, you will be all right, while if you are bleeding in early pregnancy and are not feeling nausea, then that is a very bad sign. Again, there is nothing to document these folk theories as medically sound.

Bleeding in early pregnancy

Can you have periods while you are pregnant?

Although one of the first signs of pregnancy is the absence of an expected period, as many as one third of all pregnant women will have normal bleeding in their early pregnancies, and may continue to have it for the first 3 months. Many women, in fact, bleed to such an extent that they do not know they are pregnant until the fourth or fifth month. It is these women who present themselves to their doctor with a "new" pregnancy, only to learn that their dates are wildly out of line. In the old days, when induced or therapeutic abortion was harder to come by, this would cause a woman with an unwanted pregnancy a lot of heartache; she would be told she was 5 months pregnant and beyond the legal limit for an abortion. So, if there is a chance you could be pregnant, and your monthly period appears very slight (just a couple of days and not much more than spotting), do see your doctor immediately.

Spotting is usually dark brown or very deep red in color, and it often happens around the time of your first, second, or third missed period. It happens either because the levels of progesterone and HCG are not yet high enough to suppress the period totally or, maybe, because there has been a minor fall in hormone levels as the placenta starts to take over the function of the corpus luteum in the ovary (luteo-placental shift). The bleeding is *not* from the embryo but from unoccupied areas in the uterus, so it will not harm the pregnancy. As long as the bleeding is not accompanied by cramps or periodlike pains, there is every chance nothing is wrong. It is quite a normal occurrence in early pregnancy.

Nevertheless, if you have such spotting, you should go to bed and report the bleeding to your doctor, who will examine you; (remember that a vaginal examination will not cause a miscarriage). You may also be given an ultrasound scan to make sure there is nothing abnormal, by which I mean an ectopic (tubal) pregnancy, a blighted ovum, or a molar pregnancy (see pages 105–106), all of which are very unlikely. However, irregular bleeding can be a symptom of any of these conditions, in which case the absence of a fetus will be detected from the ultrasound picture. But such bleeding can also result from other causes not directly related to pregnancy, such as the heavy vaginal discharge that can be symptomatic of the thrush fungus or Trichomonas.

If some slight spotting or bleeding follows intercourse, you should also tell your doctor. During pregnancy it is not uncommon for bleeding to occur from the cervix after intercourse. The cervix is engorged with blood, which is why it turns a purplish color and why, if pressed upon, there may occur some loss of blood. The doctor will examine your cervix with a speculum to see if there are any lesions or signs of trauma. Such bleeding after intercourse will not cause any problems with the pregnancy unless it is discovered that your cervix is opening, in which case intercourse must be stopped until these first 3 months of pregnancy have passed.

Why does spotting or bleeding happen in early pregnancy?

We do not know why exactly, but the cause may be hormonal. It should not harm the baby, provided your doctor conducts further tests to ensure that all is well with the pregnancy. There is no need to fear for the baby's health if you have had any such bleeding, as long as your pregnancy settles down and the hormone levels remain sufficient. The bleeding does not come from the baby, but from the uterine lining, which has not yet been occupied by the growing pregnancy. The only reported effect on babies is that sometimes they are born with slightly lower birth weight.

It is interesting to consider how dramatically things have changed in the last decade or so. In the old days if a woman bled in early pregnancy, and she went to her doctor or the hospital emergency room, a diagnosis had to rely purely on clinical judgment as to whether she had already miscarried or whether the pregnancy was still alive. Her doctor may have said "Let's scrape you out and start again." Or, she might have been made to stay in bed as a form of treatment, only to experience continued anxiety and possibly terrible disappointment if the pregnancy failed to thrive.

Fortunately the effect of such bleeding on a continuing pregnancy is no longer such a mystery, and the guesswork has largely been taken out of its management in early pregnancy because of two modern techniques. First, your doctor can measure the levels of the pregnancy hormones progesterone and HCG (and possibly another hormone, relaxin).

Second, with the help of ultrasound, the doctor can look for certain healthy signs: the position of the developing fetal sac, which should be high up in the uterus, and the presence of a fetus or fetal heart, in the sac. With these results the doctor can decide on the prognosis for your pregnancy and whether it is worth putting you to bed to try to conserve it.

Should you go to bed if you suffer slight bleeding?

If you are bleeding, it is generally a good rule to get off your feet. While you are waiting to see the doctor, and particularly if you are anxious, do stay in bed and curtail your physical activities as much as possible. I cannot say it is vital you stay in bed, though activities associated with being upright may stimulate contractions and further bleeding. As long as you are having no low abdominal pain, or back pain, and the spotting is mild, there is probably no problem.

How can you tell if you are going to miscarry?

You can bleed quite heavily in early pregnancy and not miscarry, nor will the baby be affected. As long as the bleeding is painless and does not continue for too many days, all is well. The bad signs are bleeding with pain or menstruallike cramps, because these can mean the uterus is starting to abort the fetus. If the bleeding is very heavy with large clots, then it probably will become a miscarriage. The clots have formed because there is so much blood in the vagina that it has time to coagulate.

The color of the blood you are losing is very relevant. If you bleed a little, the blood goes into the top of the vagina, where it stays for several hours while you sleep or until physical activity or pressure from going to the toilet forces it out; in which case the blood will be brown or dark red—meaning the flow is not active and not directly dangerous. If it turns red, and continues to flow fresh bright red, the bleeding is active and you should visit your doctor.

Incomplete abortion: If you have bled a lot with some pain, and then continue to have a trickle of blood, you must see your doctor. It might be that you have had an incomplete abortion, as some of the tissue of the pregnancy has remained in the uterus or the cervix. This tissue must be removed as it may cause more rapid hemorrhage at a future time, and it can become infected. Your doctor will therefore empty your uterus by the best method, which will mean a suction of the contents of the uterus either under a local or general anesthetic, depending on the stage of your pregnancy. As your cervix will have dilated to allow the passage of blood clots and pregnancy tissue (which caused your cramps), the process will not be painful, even with a local anesthetic (an injection into the cervix). Once the uterus has been emptied, you may find that you suffer further cramping. This can be relieved by aspirin, or by a strong drink (alcohol is a very good uterine relaxant—and you may feel you deserve a stiff drink by that time).

Missed abortion (retained miscarriage): Light brown bleeding accompanied by a growing awareness that you no longer "feel" pregnant (the breasts may no longer feel swollen, and the nausea has passed too quickly), could indicate that the fetus has died inside you, but has failed to abort and is still in the uterus.

In the old days it was hard for a doctor to diagnose whether the onset of the bleeding was a threatened miscarriage that had now settled, or a missed abortion in which the fetus was no longer growing. These days, however, using ultrasound, your doctor will be able to locate the empty sac in the uterus and give you a swift and definite answer.

If you have suffered this emotionally painful condition, you may prefer to go into the hospital and have the remains of the pregnancy removed by D & C, rather than wait for your body to expel the fetus and its sac in its own good time.

Although this is a harrowing situation, at least with ultrasound the emergency is taken out of it. You will not have to wait and worry about miscarriage, and that should help lessen any guilt you are feeling about the fetus dying inside you.

Do not assume future pregnancies will follow this pattern, as the recurrence rate is low. If there is a repeated miscarriage, your doctor may send tissue from the pregnancy to a genetics laboratory for examination and investigation for chromosomal abnormalities. However, many genetics laboratories require that at least three consecutive miscarriages have taken place before they undertake expensive chromosomal testing, as the chance of finding a chromosomal abnormality is very low.

What if you do miscarry?

If you begin to bleed slowly at first, but then find the volume increasing and the flow heavy with clots; if the bleeding is associated with low abdominal pain, or menstrual-type cramps, particularly if the pain becomes severe; you should contact your doctor immediately, or go directly to the nearest emergency room.

Even if the blood is coming out in large clots, do not panic. It forms clots because, as it builds up volume in the vagina, it coagulates before emission. Do *not* use a tampon to control the flow, as this can either lead to infection getting into the uterus or bring on yet more bleeding. The pain you are suffering is not an indication of some terrible catastrophe, but simply that uterine contractions have started and the body is readying itself to abort the fetus. A miscarriage is very similar to labor, except you have none of the excitement of the climax to look forward to. It is inevitably distressing, but it can be made worse if you fear you are going to bleed to death—which you will not.

Women do not die from miscarriages, nor do they bleed to death. You are not hemorrhaging, but dispelling all the uterine blood and tissue built up during the weeks of the pregnancy. Even if you start to bleed during the night, unless the bleeding is excessive or you have very severe contractions, there is no need to contact your doctor until the morning. If the bleeding is heavy or you have pain, you can always go to the emergency room first, and then contact your doctor.

Sometimes I am asked if there is a hormone treatment that will prevent such miscarriages. Basically there is no way of stopping an inevitable miscarriage once there is cramping and heavy bleeding. Hormonal measurement was only introduced in the early 1970s, so the hormone treatments that were given in the past were generally inaccurately used, often with harmful effects. Because it is very hard to know whether the miscarriage has been caused by low hormone levels, or whether the fetus has already died and this has led to the reduction in hormones, it is virtually impossible to assess whether the pregnancy could be saved.

What other "false" positives can occur in early pregnancy?

Blighted ovum is probably the cause of many early miscarriages. Precisely what happens is uncertain. You have all the normal conditions of pregnancy, including missing a period and a positive pregnancy test, but the pregnancy fails to develop a fetus. For about 6 weeks, the so-called conception carries on as normal: it implants in the uterus and the corpus luteum produces hormones that suppress the periods—but no fetus grows, only other pregnancy tissue.

A woman may have suspicions about the normality of this "pregnancy," particularly if she has been pregnant before. She will have none of the usual nausea, breast swelling, tingling of the nipples, alterations of taste or sleepiness. She might say "I just don't feel pregnant." Eventually, between 8 and 10 weeks after "conception," she will start to bleed, probably a slow trickle of brown discolored blood, gradually increasing into a steady flow. She will fear a miscarriage and should contact her doctor. In the end, the contents of the uterus will come out, as if she were having a very heavy period. The doctor will need to examine her once the bleeding begins, to determine whether all the tissue from the uterus has been evacuated. The evacuation may need to be completed in the office by the aspiration method, or the patient may have to be hospitalized overnight for a D & C. The end result is like a minor early miscarriage, but it is not usually accompanied by much pain.

Ectopic pregnancy (see also page 16): Sometimes the fertilized ovum takes too long to travel down the Fallopian tube. On the seventh day, instead of reaching the uterus and implanting there, it will embed itself in the Fallopian tube and there the beginnings of a pregnancy will occur. Pregnancy hormones are produced at levels sufficient to suppress a period, and a woman can receive confirmation of pregnancy from a pregnancy test. She may not find out about her condition until her first visit to the doctor, when, on internal examination, the physician will find that the uterus has not expanded as in a normal pregnancy. The patient will then be examined by ultrasound to support these findings.

With an ectopic (tubal) pregnancy, it is unlikely you would suffer the nausea associated with early pregnancy, but you will begin to experience low abdominal cramping, maybe some slight spotting or staining of very dark blood, some dizziness or shoulder-tip pain. If such pains begin or bleeding increases, you must get to your doctor or the hospital emergency room as quickly as possible, as rupture of the tube can be extremely dangerous to your life or to your future fertility. With early treatment, however, the pregnancy may be removed and the tube can often be repaired. So, if you should suffer a missed period (or very scanty dark spotting), associated with low abdominal pain, do see your doctor as soon as possible to investigate for this condition.

When would ultrasound be used in early pregnancy?

For all women, perhaps, the biggest frustration in pregnancy is that they cannot see inside themselves to watch the developing baby, or to check that it is all right. When you lose blood, suffer excessive vomiting, or feel no nausea, the tendency is to panic and assume that something must be wrong. You can imagine, therefore, how difficult it used to be when obstetricians could only rely on clinical judgment in assessing what was actually happening and how best to advise the patient.

The clinical signs of a pregnancy include a bluish or violet discoloration of the vagina, softening of the cervix, and slight enlargement of the uterus. These signs may not tell the doctor too much more at this stage. Questions such as whether the pregnancy is normally located in the uterus or implanted elsewhere, and whether the fetus is actually alive, may be difficult to answer. Fetal parts cannot be felt until the twenty-sixth week. With a stethoscope, fetal heart sounds can be heard at the eighteenth week. These days, however, with ultrasonic fetal heartbeat monitoring (Fetone), the baby's heartbeat can be picked up and heard by the doctor and mother at 9 to 10 weeks of pregnancy (7 to 8 weeks of fetal life). Certainly the rapid flutter of the tiny drumlike beats (160 to 180 times a minute in early pregnancy) is the most welcome sound for all concerned. Hearing the fetal heart means the pregnancy is alive and correctly placed. Seeing an image of the fetus itself provides even more answers.

Ultrasound (ultrasonography) uses sound waves that pass into the body and that reflect off solid material within the body. These waves are in turn transmitted onto a screen that is rather like a TV screen. Using ultrasound between 6 and 8 weeks of pregnancy, your doctor can diagnose a viable pregnancy, an ectopic (tubal) pregnancy, a molar pregnancy, a blighted ovum, or a miscarriage, all by looking for the fetal sac, noting its position, and watching for a fetal heart or fetal motion. Early ultrasound, by the way, will also detect a twin or multiple birth more efficiently and far in advance of previous diagnostic ability. Whether pregnancy ultrasound should be routine for all pregnancies, to detect any abnormalities, is still being debated and is a very controversial question.

Ultrasound was developed because of the desire to find a safe alternative to the use of X rays for early diagnosis of pregnancy, since X rays can harm the fetus. X rays show only bony structures, such as the fetal spine, from the seventeenth week of pregnancy at the earliest. So compared to ultrasound, X rays are not even very efficient. Ultrasound has now been in use for about 15 years and there have been no documented reports of any problems. Repeat scans are safe if necessary.

It has been generally agreed that the benefits of ultrasound

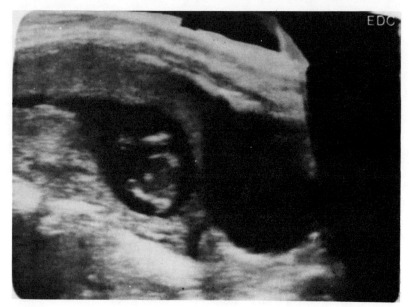

FIG. A.

FIG. B.

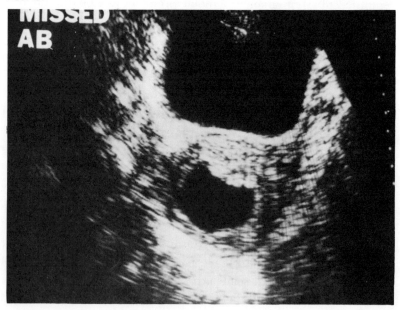

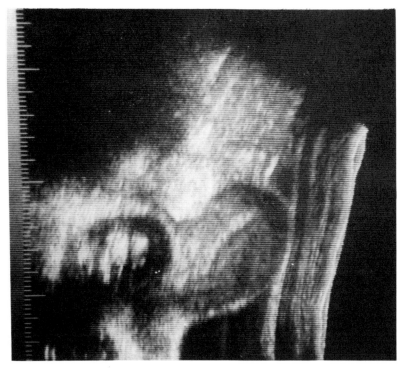

FIG. C.

Ultrasound pictures taken in early pregnancy help your doctor make an accurate assessment of the pregnancy, or of related conditions as early as 8–10 weeks.

FIG. A. This is a normal pregnancy at 8–9 weeks. You can see, at top, the abdominal wall of the mother and then the baby's head in the uterus.

FIG. B. A missed abortion. This time the uterus, with an *empty* amniotic sac inside, is visible.

FIG. C. A tubal pregnancy. The picture shows the abdominal wall and uterus. However, the uterus is empty and there is a fetal head outside, implanted in the Fallopian tube.

Slides courtesy of Yale University Medical School, Dept. of Ob/Gyn, Perinatal Unit.

far outweigh any possible consequences. However, as in all such cases, the cost/benefit ratio has to be determined by mother and obstetrician. And as with any procedure in medicine, it must only be used when indicated. (For a further discussion on ultrasound, its technology, and whether you can choose not to have such an examination, see pages 193–194.)

YOU AND YOUR OBSTETRICIAN

How to choose your doctor

If you do not already have a gynecologist or obstetrician whom you like and trust for childbirth, then no doubt you will ask friends or relatives to suggest someone compatible with your views of pregnancy and labor. The only criterion for judging the doctor's professional ability is that he or she should be a board-certified member of the American College of Obstetricians and Gynecologists (ACOG). It is an added credit if he or she is affiliated with a teaching institution. If that is the case, you can be sure your doctor is up to date.

How are you to know if the doctor is competent? The ACOG membership should be a sufficient recommendation. Otherwise, you can go on a personal recommendation from an internist or from your family doctor. You could telephone the nearby teaching hospital, ask for a list of their staff, and find out whom they recommend most. If you are new to the area, maybe your best course would be to ask your previous doctor for a recommendation in the new area. Most doctors have a professional network of colleagues and know who is doing well in certain fields.

You may wish to meet the doctor for a brief interview before committing yourself. Discuss the question of fees, of course, and methods of payment. Make it clear what type of labor process you would prefer, because if you are definitely interested in natural childbirth or any special procedure, you will need a doctor sympathetic to your attitude. You should also be thinking "Is this doctor prepared to listen to my anxieties, and to give me time and compassion, as well as expertise?"

If there is not a well-trained specialist in your area, you may of course have your pregnancy managed by a general practitioner, who may also deliver the baby. But if you fall into any high-risk category, you should be seen by a specialist in the nearest teaching hospital.

How can you tell if you are high-risk and need a specialist?

If you are a teenager under eighteen; an adult of advanced maternal age (thirty-five or over, in any pregnancy); if you have had two or more spontaneous miscarriages; have had a previous stillbirth or neonatal death; if you have had a premature baby; suffer from diabetes, heart disease, or high blood pressure; have had a caesarean section; or have had a previous abnormal baby, then you are considered high-risk.

When should you first see your doctor in pregnancy?

If you miss a period and know you could be pregnant, then see your doctor when you are just a few days overdue so you can have the pregnancy blood test and a confirmation one way or the other as soon as possible.

Right from the beginning you will want to discuss with your doctor questions such as nutrition, vitamins, rest, and anything pressing on your mind.

Although you may not really "feel" pregnant, if you have read the first chapter of this book, you will be aware how very important it is to be careful what you take into the body—no medical drugs, social drugs, over-the-counter remedies, alcohol, cigarettes, caffeine, even air pollutants if you can possibly avoid them—in these very early weeks.

The importance of regular visits

Many women are careless about making regular visits. Yet pregnancy is a wonderful time to practice preventive medicine; after all, you are not ill, and there is no need to become ill. Your prenatal visits are of the utmost importance. Pregnancy lasts 40 weeks (280 days) and your visits allow detection at the very start of any complications. Prenatal care is actually as important as labor and delivery.

Good prenatal care and the use of the new techniques I am describing in this book make pregnancy and childbirth a safe and worry-free experience—if the doctor is given a chance to use them.

From the time pregnancy is diagnosed, regular visits are made usually every 4 weeks until the thirty-second week of pregnancy, every 2 weeks from the thirty-second to the thirty-sixth week and, for the final month, every week. This plan is modified according to the physician's interpretation of a patient's needs, and many doctors keep the visits to 3 weeks apart.

Do not neglect the rapport between you and your doctor on the visits. And, if you feel you are not being given enough time, or if the doctor rushes you instead of listening to your questions and anxieties, do not be afraid to change doctors in midpregnancy. It will not harm the baby, and it might well improve your labor. Patients in the 1980s must not be afraid to speak their feelings to their doctors. You should be working as a team. In order to guide, help, and support you in this particular physical condition, the physician needs your trust and confidence. If you do not get along well with your doctor, it could lead to problems in labor, as you may suffer from a special form of tension in trying to "perform" for this uncompassionate person.

How does the doctor know when you will be due?

The average pregnancy lasts 266 days after ovulation, which occurs about 2 weeks after the first day of your last period (so pregnancy lasts 280 days in all). This is still a very rough estimate and there is a wide range of normal delivery dates. The way to work out your due date is to add 7 days to the first day of your last normal period, subtract 3 months, and add 1 year. So, if your last period began on April 17, 1982, your due date will be January 24, 1983. Because pregnancy can vary so much in length, in fact only about 60 percent of patients deliver within a week of this calculation, and only 5 percent on the actual date. We generally let patients go up to 2 weeks past their due date, before considering inducing the birth.

What does the doctor do on your first visit—and why?

The first visit to your doctor will be the longest. Called the "booking visit," it is always more detailed and time-consuming than follow-up visits. The first step is the taking and recording of a careful medical history. The doctor asks you for some of the information I have mentioned earlier in the book, about your medical and surgical background. It is best, even if it seems an undue waste of time, for the doctor to write notes as you talk, rather than to hand you a form to fill in, as this way he or she can prod your memory to make sure all the necessary details are included.

You will be asked your age, and your husband's age (relevant if he is over fifty-five), how long you have been married, what your line of work is, what form of contraception you have used, about your family's medical history, whether there are any familial diseases, such as diabetes, which may become highlighted in pregnancy; any twins or triplets in the family; all about your previous pregnancies, prenatal complications, the deliveries, miscarriages, or abortions. Do not hide any miscarriages or abortions from your doctor, as they are relevant to your care and the information will be treated with confidence.

The doctor will ask about this current pregnancy, and inquire about complications such as any bleeding, nausea, or excessive vomiting.

Then it will be time for a general physical examination. You will be *weighed* to establish what we call the "baseline weight," from which it can be seen whether you gain too much or too little in the course of the pregnancy. The reason for this caution about weight, as you will read later in this chapter, is that there is a normal optimal weight gain that is within the area of 25 to 30 pounds by the end of the pregnancy. Your weight gain has an effect on the baby's birth weight and on your own health during and after the pregnancy.

Your *blood pressure* will be checked, because any subsequent rise must be assessed as it could lead to complications. Pre-eclampsia is one of the causes of a raised blood pressure in pregnancy. It is peculiar to pregnancy and means not only a raised blood pressure but some body swelling (edema), and that you will be passing protein into your urine. It clears up between pregnancies and, if detected and treated, it should have no harmful effects on you or your baby. Your doctor will be so concerned to detect and treat pre-eclampsia that he or she will take your blood pressure reading at every visit. If you do have a raised blood pressure at any point, the cause will be investigated, and some form of treatment will be advised.

The physical examination begins with a general checkup, going through your body's major systems. The doctor listens to your heart and lungs, checks your thyroid and breasts for lumps or abnormalities, and checks your abdomen for any obvious abnormalities.

The doctor will make various maneuvers with his or her hands to feel the height of the uterus in the abdomen, in order to check the stage of your pregnancy and the position of the baby.

At such an early stage, it is not significant whether the baby is lying head down or up, for the size of the fetus relative to the amount of amniotic fluid means the baby constantly floats around and changes position. Your doctor will also assess whether the size of the baby relates to your dates, and how much amniotic fluid there is. Your physician can also feel if the uterus is irritable: if it contracts each time it is touched, it may be a sign of some growth retardation (that the baby is not receiving sufficient nutrition from the placenta).

The doctor listens to the fetal heart, often with the help of a piece of electronic equipment called a Fetone.

From there, the doctor proceeds to the pelvic, or internal, examination. It is important that you understand that an internal in early pregnancy is not a dangerous procedure. It will not set off a miscarriage. The examination does produce some very vital findings. For example, any infections such as a fungus will be found and a Pap smear can be taken to ensure that the cervix is healthy. The doctor can also assess the length of the cervix to see whether it is incompetent or weak. The size of the uterus will be assessed and the doctor can reassure you that there is not a tubal (ectopic) pregnancy. The doctor will also be able to exclude tumors of the ovaries. If any such tumors are found they will be treated, since they can obstruct labor or delivery. (They are, however, very rare.)

Pelvic assessment, or measurement, is not done so early in pregnancy, because the size of the baby cannot yet be anticipated. Whether you have a six- or a ten-pound baby inside will make all the difference. Also, your bones will relax slightly later in pregnancy, and the size of your pelvis will increase.

During the internal, your doctor takes a culture for gonorrhea by placing a swab in the vagina. The disease may have occurred years ago and will not harm the baby unless it is in your vagina at the time of delivery. But, as gonorrhea is so common now, many doctors feel it worth the routine check.

What does it mean if your uterus lies backward (retroverted)?

During the internal examination your doctor may determine whether your uterus lies backward. This position is found in about 20 percent of women and means nothing more than that it is tilted back. This is quite normal and will have no effect on the pregnancy. It is, however, useful for the doctor to know about because, when the uterus fills the pelvis, at about 12 weeks, it then swings forward into a position in which it can grow normally. If your uterus does not swing forward, the doctor will discover this on a repeat internal examination at 12 weeks, and will maneuver it painlessly with his or her hands.

What are the other tests at your first visit to the doctor?

At the first visit (and all subsequent ones) a small amount of your urine will be tested with a dip stick. Some doctors let you pass the urine in the office; others ask you to bring a specimen. No jam jars please!

The urine is tested first for sugar. However, the presence of sugar in the urine is not enough to cause concern, as your kidneys may pass sugar into the urine during pregnancy though your blood sugar levels are normal. But if it shows up on more than one occasion, you will be sent to a laboratory for a glucose tolerance test, which is a diabetes test that is administered over a period of 2 or 3 hours. Second, urine is tested for the presence of protein. A positive result may indicate the onset of preeclampsia, or of an infection (cystitis), or it could mean an underlying kidney disorder.

Your blood will be drawn on the first visit for several investigations. First, a blood count is done to see if you are anemic. This is often repeated at about the thirty-second week of pregnancy. Women need iron supplementation in pregnancy, for not only is the demand increased by the baby, but the extra blood circulating dilutes the proportion of iron in your blood.

Anemia must be guarded against because, aside from making the mother very tired, it can lead to premature labor and a small baby. A screening test for syphilis known as the VDRL (Venereal Disease Research Laboratory) test will also be done on the blood (see page 48).

Some doctors have the blood tested for viral diseases as well. This kind of testing is very new, so do not expect it as a routine part of prenatal care. The tests are known collectively as the TORCH titers, referring to the viruses investigated: Toxoplasmosis, Rubella (German measles), Chlamydia and Herpes (see pages 25–26). If a pregnant woman contracts a viral infection during her pregnancy, it is very hard to assess its nature since everyone has some degree of viral antibodies in the blood left over from previous viral diseases (e.g., measles). If your own baseline of these infections has been established, should you become reexposed to a viral illness during pregnancy, your doctor will have a rising level with which to compare.

In certain areas, primarily for black populations, sickle-cell anemia (see pages 189–190) screening is also done at the first doctor's visit.

Subsequent prenatal visits are not so detailed. You are always weighed, your blood pressure is taken, the uterus is palpated, and the urine is tested. Any problems you encounter, or anxieties you are suffering, should be discussed with your doctor.

Ultrasound is done by some doctors as a routine screening in all pregnancies, to check for any abnormalities, determine the maturity of the infant, and to monitor its growth. Other doctors, however, will only do an ultrasound scan when specific information is required (see pages 106–110, 192–193, for information on ultrasound in the first and second trimesters). Whether ultrasound should become part of routine prenatal care is still being debated. The role of the screening process has not yet been fully established, nor has it been decided whether it would be economically beneficial to give every pregnant woman an ultrasound scan. But a decision will have to be made very soon. As yet, however, your doctor is under no legal or medical pressure to give you an ultrasound scan unless it appears to be necessary.

Blood grouping and the Rh factor

Your blood type is determined at the first visit to your obstetrician. It is very important to discover whether you belong to blood groups A, B, AB or O in case you need a transfusion at delivery—but even more important is to discover the Rh grouping you fall into.

Most people have never had to consider whether they are what is known as Rh negative or Rh positive, until they become pregnant. The Rh factor is a condition of the blood affecting us all, one that has a potentially unique and specific harmful effect for the pregnant woman if she belongs to one group and her husband to the other.

The majority of women are Rh positive. In fact, 85 percent of white women and a higher proportion of black and Oriental women are Rh positive. For those 15 percent who are Rh negative, their husband's blood must also be tested. If the husband happens to be Rh negative as well, there will be no problem. But if he is Rh Positive, then the woman's pregnancy may run into complications.

When incompatible blood groups are mixed, the recipient's body develops antibodies to the "foreign" blood type. This can occur during a blood transfusion for an operation or accident, or when you become pregnant.

The Rh factor is so called because it was first discovered in the blood of Rhesus monkeys. Basically, the blood cells of each person contain six factors, three inherited from the mother and three from the father. Each blood group is Rh positive or Rh negative, no matter which combination of the factors is inherited. The only one that is significant is known as the "big D," the dominant gene. If you possess one "big D" (the positive factor) and one "little d" (the negative factor) then your blood will still be positive. But if a man's blood is "big D" (positive) and his wife's is "little d" (negative), their child's blood will be positive—which is where the problem in pregnancy may arise: the mother will be carrying a fetus which has a different Rh factor from her own.

Fetal blood cells inevitably pass into the maternal circulation, and when they do, the mother's blood produces antibodies to the fetal blood cells (containing the foreign antigen "big D"). The antibodies cross into the fetal circulation and kill off the baby's red blood cells so it becomes very anemic. Usually the baby is born prematurely and severely lacking in oxygen (a condition that gave rise to the term "blue baby") and is in need of an immediate transfusion. This disease, known as hemolytic disease of the newborn, used to be a big killer of babies, either in the womb or just after birth. Today, however, it has been virtually eradicated.

You are at greatest risk of receiving fetal blood just after birth, since this is the time of its maximal passage into your circulation. However, it has been shown that because of certain procedures, this transfusion of blood from the fetus to you may occur prenatally (see page 121).

Generally speaking, even with such a mix of blood types the first pregnancy passes without incident, as the antibodies that are formed are not sufficient to destroy the positive cells of the baby. These antibodies in the mother's blood will remain in her body, however, and Rh disease is most likely to occur in a subsequent pregnancy.

How is Rh disease controlled?

In the early 1960s, some quarter century after the Rh factor was first discovered, scientists discovered Rhogam, a drug that kills the baby's Rh-positive cells that have entered the blood of the Rh-negative woman, preventing her from producing anti-bodies in response to the presence of positive cells. This exciting development has meant that one disease has almost been wiped out—except in those few cases caused by human error when the incompatibility is not recognized and Rhogam is not given.

Rhogam should be given to an Rh-negative mother within 72 hours of birth, before her body becomes sensitized and when the drug cannot harm the baby. Rhogam eradicates the Rh factor in the mother's blood and prevents the formation of antibodies. The next pregnancy can start afresh with no problems. Similarly, Rhogam should be given after a miscarriage or abortion, or if the mother has an amniocentesis or has an external cephalic version of her baby (the baby is turned from a breech to a head presentation via abdominal pressure). There is even a move now being evaluated by the American College of Obstetricians and Gynecologists to give Rhogam to all Rh-negative mothers at about the thirtieth week of pregnancy, in order to further stamp out the disease once and for all.

How can Rhogam be administered after amniocentesis if we are not yet entirely certain of its effect on the fetus? This is a case of the benefit of medication outweighing the risk involved. The needle for the amniocentesis might enter the placenta, which would promote a mixing of the two blood types and so cause sensitization. The dose of Rhogam given after amniocentesis is much smaller than that given after birth.

If you already have Rh disease from a previous untreated pregnancy or from a blood transfusion, then Rhogam will not be able to help you. Your pregnancy will have to be very carefully managed, and should be monitored in a large perinatal center. The level of antibodies in your bloodstream will be measured at stages throughout the pregnancy, and you will probably be given an amniocentesis to see how badly affected the fetus is. If the baby is suffering from red-blood-cell destruction, this will show up in the amniotic fluid as an elevated level of bilirubin. If there appears to be a serious problem, and the baby is too immature to be delivered, then a blood transfusion may be given to the baby, while it is still in the uterus. Intra-uterine transfusion is quite a new technique and will be per-formed by a trained specialist. It lasts about an hour and can be repeated every 2 weeks. There is a 15 percent mortality rate for the baby, but without the transfusion the baby would surely die.

Jaundice in the newborn can be a symptom of the milder forms of Rh disease. The baby goes yellow, due to bilirubin pigment in the blood. If the level of bilirubin gets too high, the baby will be put under very bright lights with dark pads over its eyes. This can look alarming to the new parent, but the lights will not harm the baby as long as the eyes are pro-tected. The bright light actually breaks down the bilirubin, en-abling the baby's body to eliminate it more rapidly.

If the level of bilirubin is dangerously high, an exchange blood transfusion can be done after the birth, through the baby's um-bilical cord, which rapidly removes the yellow pigment and prevents possible brain damage.

The mother can also be sensitive to other blood types. If, for example, her blood is group O and the fetus has group A or B, she can become sensitized in a milder but similar way. This is one of the commonest causes of newborn jaundice. Even with-out incompatible blood groups, the baby may turn slightly yel-low on the second or third day after birth (see page 288). This jaundice happens because the extra blood cells picked up in intrauterine life are now breaking down, releasing the yellow bilirubin pigment. It is transient and has usually gone by the time you are ready to leave the hospital.

WEIGHT GAIN AND NUTRITION

A few simple rules should help direct you through this controversial area of obstetrics. Each doctor seems to have his or her own opinion, and many women appear confused.

1) Do not go on any diets, fad or otherwise, while you are pregnant. It is dangerous to reduce your caloric intake. This "starvation" causes the body to break down retained fats for energy, thus creating fatty acids, called ketones, that can cross the placenta and may harm the baby. 2) Try to eat whole-wheat bread, green and yellow leafy vegetables, and increase your intake of protein (meat and fish) slightly so the baby has adequate protein for its growth. Proteins are most important in pregnancy. 3) Do not skip meals. Try to eat lightly but well, regularly throughout the day, so your blood sugar level never goes down precipitously. For a well-balanced and nutritious diet, eat a full breakfast of maybe an egg and toast, or cereal and juice; a lunch of salad, with tuna or chicken; and a dinner of fish or meat, vegetables, and salad. 4) Cut down on cakes, cookies, ice cream, and sugar-containing desserts. 5) Do not drink alcohol, and limit your consumption of coffee or caffeine-containing drinks to no more than *three* such drinks a day. 6) If you become constipated, ensure an adequate fluid intake (water, fruit juices) and sufficient roughage in the form of bran, raw fruits, or cereals.

It was once thought that the baby would always take from the mother what it needed, no matter what she ate. However, it is now understood that the baby can become undernourished in the uterus, and that the mother's diet must be adequate in amount and substance; and that protein is especially important.

You will probably feel hungrier, particularly after the first trimester has passed, and you may eat larger meals than was your custom, without gaining excessive weight. But be careful not to indulge the ever-growing waistline with cakes, sodas, and ice cream. Many pregnant women seem to get a craving for sweet things, which may be hormonally induced, but should not be indulged. Do not use the excuse that you are eating for two.

What is the optimal weight gain you should aim for?

Generally, your optimal weight gain should be about 25 pounds; you should not gain any less than 15 pounds or more than 30 pounds. The reason for the under and over marks is that if you gain more than 30 pounds you might bring out some diabetic tendencies; further, the extra weight will make you feel uncomfortable, the pregnancy less pleasurable, and will be hard to lose after pregnancy. On the other hand, if you gain too little weight, it could lead to deficiencies in the baby, and to a low birth weight (known as intrauterine growth retardation, IUGR).

What is the weight gain made up of? The uterus will eventually weigh about 2 pounds, the breasts 1 extra pound, extra blood 2 pounds, body fluids in your tissue 2 pounds, and extra fat about 8 pounds—which totals 15 pounds. The extra weight you gain from the baby totals around 9½ pounds (more if the baby is heavy), broken down as follows: the baby weighs an average 6½ pounds, the placenta about 1½ pounds, and the amniotic fluid about 1½ pounds. So the combined weight gain comes to around 24½ pounds. Anything more is probably fat and extra fluid.

In the first trimester, you should gain no more than 3 pounds because the baby has not started to put on any fat. Then, for the remaining 28 weeks you should gain about three quarters of a pound a week, in all about 21 pounds, for a total of 24 pounds. I will break that down into a chart so you can check your own weight gain.

In the first 20 weeks, altogether you should gain about 8 pounds; and from 20 weeks on you should double the amount of weight gained. As a rough guide, therefore, from 20 to 40 weeks you should be gaining at the most 1 pound a week, and

TIME	USUAL GAIN ON AN ADEQUATE DIET
0–12 weeks	2 lbs.
12–16 weeks	2 lbs.
17–20 weeks	4 lbs.
21–24 weeks	4 lbs.
25–28 weeks	4 lbs.
29–32 weeks	3 lbs.
33–36 weeks	3 lbs.
36–40 weeks	2 lbs.
Total	24 lbs.

before that the rate should be much slower—around half a pound or less a week.

Most women can afford to gain a little more every now and again, as nature exerts its own balances. For example, you may not have your first weigh-in with the obstetrician at the booking visit until you are already 6 weeks pregnant, yet there will be little cause for concern if you gain over 24 pounds in the remainder of the pregnancy. Toward the end of the pregnancy, in the last week or so, your weight may even go down as the amniotic fluid decreases and the reproductive changes are readying themselves for birth. But do try to limit yourself and remember that any more than 2 pounds a week, at any stage of the pregnancy, is regarded as excessive. Your obstetrician has to be careful to note any rapid gain in weight, for it might also be a sign that you are retaining body fluid (which could be a symptom of pre-eclampsia which would be dangerous to you and the baby). Your doctor will not complain about your excessive weight gain for vanity's sake, nor to give you a hard time. It is for strict medical reasons that your weight gain must be observed.

If you are going to weigh yourself, as well as be weighed by your doctor at the visits, make sure to do it at the same time each day, wearing the same clothes, so you can properly judge weight fluctuations.

When you see your doctor at the booking visit, if you weigh under 100 pounds or over 200 pounds either extreme will be very significant to the management of your pregnancy.

Weight loss at any stage of the pregnancy may be of significance to the doctor as it could be a sign of placental insufficiency (the placenta may be failing in its function of transporting food and oxygen from the mother to the baby) leading to fetal starvation. In early pregnancy, however, weight loss is usually because the mother is nauseated and she, not the baby, is losing the weight.

Is there any help for controlling your weight?

If you are gaining too rapidly in pregnancy, you will have to discuss nutrition and exercise with your doctor in an effort to control it. Remember, never put yourself on a diet in an attempt to lose weight. Your baby needs you to eat. But it does not need junk food, excess carbohydrates, or gallons of soda in your, or its, system.

Much of the weight control will be up to you, and it may depend on how active you remain through pregnancy and whether you take some form of regular exercise (see pages 50–52).

Diet pills of any kind (the ones containing amphetamines have now been banned in some states) should *never* be taken during pregnancy. They can quite easily harm the baby. Diuretics, for taking off excess body fluids, must also *never* be used in pregnancy, as they disturb the body's chemical balance and this, too, can harm the baby. It used to be thought that dieting could safely begin after the birth, but that is no longer accepted, for adequate nutrition is as important during the period of lactation as during pregnancy (see page 301).

Low-salt diets are only recommended if you are hypertensive, when high blood pressure is associated with fluid retention. Usually this just means not adding salt to your food. Unless medically advised, it is not a good idea to omit salt completely because it is vital to you and your baby, and the bland taste of unsalted food might deter you from a healthy diet.

I am often asked about the protein requirement in pregnancy. Protein is very important to the baby, but the amount you need in pregnancy is sometimes overemphasized. You will need some extra protein in pregnancy, but only about 2 pounds throughout the *whole* pregnancy over and above the amount in a normal adequate diet. Divide that by 280 days and see how small the daily requirement really is!

Milk also has been overemphasized as a necessity in pregnancy. If you have a well-balanced diet and take a vitamin supplement, then 1 additional cup of milk a day is all that is necessary. The traditional daily quart of milk that pregnant women are often advised to drink, or dairy products in the form of cheese and yogurt to make up that amount, is actually excessive and quite intolerable. You will be getting the minerals milk provides elsewhere in your diet and, if you drink so much milk, excess weight gain is inevitable.

The calcium level of the pregnant woman may decline dramatically, which is why it used to be thought that milk, a great calcium provider, should be taken in excessive amounts. But now we know that the drop in the calcium level is a normal physiological change of pregnancy and not a sign of a serious deficiency that could harm the baby. If you take vitamin supplements containing calcium you will be well covered.

If you are concerned about gaining weight, another area over which you can exert control is your fluid intake. Many people today depend on sodas to support them through the day. But I am afraid you will have to cut down on sodas. Many sodas contain caffeine, which limits their consumption. Ordinary sodas still contain too much sugar, and diet sodas contain cyclamates or saccharin, both of which might harm the fetus, though no definite evidence of this exists. Fruit juices or plain water are the safest drinks in pregnancy. Both will supply you with fluid and minerals. Fruit juices do contain a lot of fructose (natural sugar found in fruit) and you may prefer to water them down so you feed your craving and your thirst, but not your waistline.

Do you need vitamin supplements?

With a well-balanced diet, vitamin supplementation is not absolutely necessary. But the supplements specially prepared for maternal use are quite safe. Their use is optional, however, and your obstetrician has not let you down by not recommending them.

You will need iron supplementation, though, throughout pregnancy and for 3 months after birth, particularly if you are breast-feeding, as you can easily become iron deficient or anemic. The body's iron content falls in pregnancy, though there is controversy over whether this is a true deficiency or due to the increased amount of blood in circulation that dilutes the proportion of iron by volume.

Folic acid is necessary along with iron (it helps the iron be absorbed and helps build up fetal tissues). It is found naturally in liver, grains, and leafy green vegetables. But it is probably advisable to take as much as a 1-milligram tablet per day, since in some areas of the country the soil is low in folic acid, or you may not have access to the very fresh vegetables that contain the vitamin. If you are on anticonvulsant drugs for epilepsy, have a multiple pregnancy, if your diet is very poor, or you suffer from a blood disorder, then you *must* have a folic acid supplement.

As for Vitamins A, D, and C—if your diet is well-balanced, contains fresh fruits and vegetables, protein and some milk, these vitamin supplements are probably not necessary. But if you do use them, be sure to avoid an excess intake. Excesses of Vitamins C, D, and A can lead to problems in the fetus. These problems are rare but are well reported. You should never self-prescribe megavitamins during pregnancy. Just take the supplement your doctor recommends and your diet and body will take care of the rest.

How much coffee and tea can you drink?

Studies of the effects of coffee on the unborn have shown that fetal abnormalities have developed in rats given excessive quantities of this form of caffeine. But to induce an equivalent effect in a human baby, the mother would have to drink as much as 28 cups of coffee daily. There is, however, some concern about the effect of coffee during pregnancy, and you should contain your consumption to three cups of tea or coffee a day. If you drink sodas containing caffeine, you should fit your consumption of them within this limit.

May you eat junk food?

If you are determined to eat fast foods or junk foods, be careful of totally synthetic foods, such as nondairy creams. There is no proof yet that they can harm the baby, but if the foodstuff is not good for you, it certainly is not good for the baby. If you have a sweet tooth, bake some fruit pies for yourself. Try to cut down on sugary substances during pregnancy.

THE MOTHER'S HEALTH AND CONDITION

Pregnancy is not a disease, nor should it be viewed as such. Most prenatal care is preventive. You will be tested throughout the three trimesters for indications of conditions known to harm a pregnancy. If a problem is discovered, it can be treated as soon as the symptoms appear rather than after the condition has progressed.

If you suffer from epilepsy, diabetes, heart disease, or asthma, or have been treated for cancer, or are undergoing treatment for thyroid disease or high blood pressure, I advise you to look back to Chapter 1 (pages 3–84), where I dealt in detail with the management of these conditions during pregnancy.

Blood pressure testing: Your blood pressure will not usually rise above the normal level during the first trimester, unless you had high blood pressure before pregnancy, or if you have an underlying kidney disease that has not been noticed. At each visit to your doctor your blood pressure will be checked to see whether it remains within normal limits. If it does rise, it will have to be treated, as it may affect the placenta and cut down on the baby's nutritional source. This could lead to a low birth weight. Occasionally hypertension is associated with separation of the placenta from the uterine wall, an emergency situation needing vigorous treatment. However, the constant checks on the blood pressure will make the occurrence of such an emergency unlikely.

German measles (rubella): If the booking visit test shows that you have not been exposed to German measles, should you be vaccinated during pregnancy? Many women ask this question, fearing their vulnerability to the disease particularly if they work with young children who might carry the infection. *The answer is a definite no.* You have to have been vaccinated before conception, as the German measles vaccine has a weakened but live virus and may be dangerous to a fetus.

In the first 12 weeks of pregnancy, you must try to avoid contact with any child who has a high fever, even if the fever is not thought to be caused by German measles. If you have small children, there is obviously not much you can do to keep away from them, but if you are a schoolteacher I advise you to be strict about sending any feverish child straight home.

The next question is, What should you do if you come into contact with someone who has, or is suspected of having, German measles? Tell your doctor immediately, and he or she will take a blood sample, which will be sent to a laboratory for antibody testing to rubella. The test will be repeated in 10 days. Any marked rise in the level of antibodies is highly suspicious and demands a more specific test on a third blood sample. Should this test result in a suggestion you have had rubella, you and your husband will have to face the decision of whether to abort the pregnancy at this point. In early pregnancy, there is an 85 percent risk that rubella may cause some major abnormality in your child, such as blindness, heart disease, or limb defects.

I am sometimes asked about the administration of gamma globulin for a pregnant woman exposed to German measles. These are antibodies that might help, but they are very nonspecific and probably protect only the mother and not the baby. But you must discuss this with your doctor.

Cystitis: Women are often concerned that an attack of cystitis in pregnancy will harm their baby. This infection of the bladder is very common during pregnancy, particularly toward the end of the first trimester (the twelfth week is a special high-risk time) owing to changes in the urinary system. The pregnancy hormones cause dilation of the ureter and, as about 20 percent of pregnant women excrete bacteria in the urine, they are very prone to cystitis. Cystitis is not dangerous to the pregnancy unless it is associated with a prolonged high fever. If you do develop symptoms—frequent urination, burning or discomfort while you are passing urine, chills or fever—it is important to have the condition attended to. If cystitis is left untreated, it may lead to the onset of premature labor or may cause you kidney disease later in life.

Your doctor will ask for a clean-catch sample (you wash yourself and then catch the urine in midflow), and will put you on an appropriate medication while awaiting bacterial confirmation. You may be prescribed penicillin by mouth, which is safe in pregnancy. Follow-up cultures will be done after the initial treatment, to make sure the infection has been eradicated.

To guard against cystitis, you should drink an adequate amount of fluid and pay attention to hygiene.

Colds and flu: Will a cold harm the baby? This is a very common question. The answer is that a common cold does not have any effect on pregnancy, but do watch to see if you run a fever. You should bring your fever down with Tylenol (no aspirin in pregnancy) and sponging. Do not take any patent cold medicines, or those for flu that contain antihistamines (see page 31).

Influenza viruses are more virulent than those that cause common colds, especially in an Asian flu epidemic. There is some evidence that the influenza virus goes to the fetus and may cause a higher miscarriage rate. But, again, no one can be sure of its effect because a spontaneous abortion in the first trimester could have been triggered by a variety of other causes.

If you get a bad attack of flu in early pregnancy, go to your doctor, where your blood will be tested and you will be prescribed safe medication. With care and rest, the disease will pass and the pregnancy will proceed as normal.

What about vaccines against flu? The current recommendations of the U.S. Public Health Service Advisory Committee on Immunization Practices is against administering flu vaccine to pregnant women *unless* they are members of high-risk groups with cardiac or lung disease, for whom the danger of contracting flu would be greater than that associated with the vaccine itself.

Hay fever and allergies: As a general rule, during pregnancy you should not have desensitizing shots for any allergic condition because your immune system is altered and your response to the shots will be unpredictable. The required drugs are also not considered safe in pregnancy. If you are very uncomfortable, however, you may be forced to take antihistamines. Do so only on your doctor's advice, and do not use over-the-counter preparations once pregnant. Some allergic conditions improve spontaneously in pregnancy.

Mumps: If you contract mumps in pregnancy, it is usually a mild form of the disease. It will run the same course as if you were not pregnant. If you get the disease in the first 12 weeks of pregnancy, except for a minimal increase in the risk of miscarriage, there is negligible maternal and fetal risk. Mumps vaccine is contraindicated in pregnancy (as is measles vaccine) because it is live.

Chickenpox: This is an uncommon disease in adulthood and similarly uncommon in pregnancy. It can be severe if contracted, and there is a slight risk if the mother develops it shortly before delivery that the baby will develop a mild form of the chickenpox at birth. Basically, chickenpox does not cause spontaneous abortions or fetal harm.

Diarrhea: If you develop diarrhea in pregnancy, the causes and management will be the same as in nonpregnancy. Take only fluids for 24 hours and you may use Kaopectate. If there is no improvement, then consult your doctor. The condition itself will not harm the pregnancy, but if persistent, or if there is an infection in the bowel causing fever, it must be investigated and treated. For severe diarrhea, Lomotil may be prescribed; but even this will not harm the fetus.

Constipation: The condition will not harm the baby, but it does make the mother uncomfortable. A large percentage of women become constipated in pregnancy, and those who normally suffer the condition find that pregnancy aggravates it. The probable cause is the relaxant effect of the pregnancy hormone progesterone on the bowel, and in late pregnancy, the enlarged uterus also presses on the bowel and may be a factor.

Whatever the cause, it is important to prevent constipation, so make sure you have sufficient roughage in your diet. To relieve the condition, you can safely drink prune juice, eat bran cereals or whole-wheat bread, unpeeled fruits, and vegetables. You can also use a stool softener such as Colace, which is safe and may be taken as needed. Glycerine rectal suppositories are occasionally prescribed too.

It is important to remember that while the constipation itself is not a danger to pregnancy, the treatment should not be allowed to become a danger. If the constipation is severe, it is safe to use phenolphthalein or the occasional Fleet enema. Neither is it harmful to take milk of magnesia, before going to bed at night. But severe purgatives such as castor oil should be avoided, as they can induce premature labor. Mineral oil should be avoided, as it may interfere with the absorption of certain vitamins.

Flatulence: Excessive gas is common, if disturbing, in pregnancy. You may find your stomach becomes distended with gas, and that you make rather a lot of unseemly noises. Avoid large, fatty meals and gas-forming foods. Doing this, avoiding constipation, and doing regular exercises will help decrease flatulence. Heartburn or acid indigestion also affects some pregnant women, owing to the regurgitation of gastric juices. Like flatulence, heartburn will not harm the baby, but is uncomfortable to the mother. You must be careful, though, about using over-the-counter antacids. Some of them can be dangerous to the baby, particularly the ones high in salt. You may neutralize acidity with milk, Gelusil, or Maalox; both the latter two are safe and readily available antacids. Change of posture and elevating the head of the bed, at night, are helpful.

Teeth: Should you have your teeth checked in early pregnancy? Yes, because it is believed if you have any caries, they can act as a focus for bacteria, which could spread to the bloodstream. So do have a dental checkup before or during pregnancy. X rays are best postponed till after the twelfth week. If you must have X rays, your abdomen will have to be shielded, preferably with a lead shield. Some women develop more decay than usual during pregnancy for an unknown reason. Pregnancy may also promote or aggravate gum inflammation, and your dentist can advise you about any necessary additional oral hygiene.

Ideally, general anesthesia should not be given for dental

treatment in pregnancy as the agents used may affect the fetus. Local anesthesia, without Adrenalin, is safe in pregnancy if used after the twelfth week.

Minor operations: It is perfectly safe to have minor surgery during the first trimester, providing the doctor knows about the pregnancy. It is preferable to avoid a general anesthetic because it can minimize the amount of oxygen that gets to the baby. Even in emergencies, a local or regional anesthetic should be used for a pregnant woman if possible.

If the operation is to be done under local anesthetic, the amount of Adrenalin normally used can be cut down. Sometimes, it is better to wait till after the twelfth week before having the operation.

Falls: Pregnant women often fall. This is due to the enlarging abdomen altering your center of gravity, along with the weakening of all ligaments, including the ankle joints (which is a secondary hormonal effect).

Although a bad fall can be very traumatic to the pregnant woman's state of mind, such an incident rarely affects the baby and is usually not a cause for alarm. The fetus is very well cushioned within the uterus, floating in its amniotic fluid, and it could only be injured by a penetrating blow directly to the uterus. However, if you lose any blood or water after a fall, you should see your doctor immediately. Otherwise, rest quietly for a couple of hours. If afterward you notice abdominal pain or tenderness, or diminished fetal movement, contact your doctor.

Car accidents: The American Automobile Association (AAA) recommends that pregnant women wear seat belts. In later pregnancy, you may find the pressure of the shoulder belt constricting and uncomfortable, but do wear a lap belt.

Generally speaking, any injury sustained in an automobile accident will be external to you, rather than affecting the baby. There are rare cases, however, when the placenta is attached to the front wall of the uterus and an auto accident can cause abruptio placentae (separation of the placenta, see page 210). If you do receive a major blow and are feeling a lot of pain, and if there is no visible bleeding, if the uterus is tense and hard; even get to the emergency room of a hospital as soon as possible. You could have had an abruption of the placenta and not realize it.

Vaginal discharge: During pregnancy, the vagina becomes very acidic, and increases its secretions, giving a slightly acidic white discharge. A heavy discharge can be uncomfortable and distressing, particularly if you find the bed wet at night or need to wear a napkin during the day (no tampons please). But this is a normal condition of pregnancy and not one that the doctor will treat.

Any discharge found in nonpregnancy can, however, also develop in pregnancy. If you notice an itch or burning sensation, a discharge with a strong smell or a strange color, or one that is very heavy, then do report it to your doctor. For a discussion of two common fungal infections Monilia (thrush) and Trichomonas see pages 49–50.

Vaginal discharges remain localized in the vagina during pregnancy and will not affect the baby, as the mucous plug and membranes seal off the rest of the genital tract.

Gonorrhea: This can be contracted in pregnancy and result in a foul, heavy yellow discharge. It will not spread to your Fallopian tubes, as it may do in the nonpregnant state. Treatment with penicillin is used during pregnancy.

Herpes: In the first trimester of pregnancy, herpes is associated with an increase in the incidence of miscarriage (see pages 25–26). If you should contract it, go to your doctor for confirmation, which will mean taking a specimen from the lesions for culture in the laboratory. Unfortunately there is no known cure for herpes, but your doctor will be able to offer you some relief from the discomfort.

Herpes of the mouth: If herpes occurs on the lips, it is usually in the corners of the mouth and is called fever blisters or cold sores. Herpes in the mouth usually occurs on the palate, tongue, and gum tissues next to the teeth. It should be distinguished from the common canker sore, which occurs on the inside of the cheeks or lips, or in the folds of the lips. The canker sore is bacterial, not viral, but they look similar.

The herpes that affects the mouth usually is due to herpes simplex type 1. It is not as severe as genital herpes and will not affect the baby as long as it is confined to your mouth. Do not touch the vagina after you have touched your mouth. And do not indulge in fellatio, as that may infect your husband and then possibly infect your genital area. Type 1 herpes can, however, infect your genital area, as does the more usual genital type 2 virus, so you must be very careful not to contaminate your vaginal region if you have oral herpes.

Viral hepatitis (infectious hepatitis): The most common cause of jaundice in pregnant women, accounting for 50 percent of such cases, is viral hepatitis. Your skin turns yellow, as do the whites of your eyes. This can occur at any stage of pregnancy. Hepatitis B is contracted from infected needles and transfusions, and it affects the baby more severely than hepatitis A, which is an infection transmitted from the gastrointestinal tract. Hepatitis can cause the onset of premature labor and infect the baby at birth, but it is not usually associated with fetal abnormalities unless it occurs during the first trimester. It is not usually advisable to perform a therapeutic abortion. If you come into contact with someone with hepatitis A, contact your doctor immediately and have your blood tested to see if you are already infected or immune. If you are not immune to hepatitis A, you will be given an injection of gamma globulin, which is safe in pregnancy. It is not, however, a specific remedy, so it can only give you some protection rather than offer a complete cure. For hepatitis B, there is a specific antiserum, but your doctor will investigate carefully to see if you need this, as the shots are very expensive—about $400 each!

Minor complaints: Minor complaints of pregnancy may or may not cause you discomfort. We call them "minor," as they are mild conditions brought about by the physiological changes of pregnancy in the mother and they are not always treatable.

If your teeth and gums are not in excellent condition, you may suffer from bleeding gums, which can promote mouth infections. If possible, you should see your dentist before you become pregnant to help prevent this problem. Dental caries should be treated, as holes in the teeth may become a source of infection.

Nosebleeds can be worrying if frequent. They are not, however, a sign of high blood pressure. The mucous membranes lining the nasal passage have a much greater blood supply during pregnancy and a part of the nostrils may bleed very easily in pregnancy. If this occurs, gently squeeze the tip of your nose (not the bridge) between your fingers for 3 minutes. If the bleeding is persistent, an ear, nose, and throat specialist should be consulted who may cauterize the nasal vessels.

If you suffer from nasal congestion, you may use some nose drops, but do consult your doctor before using nasal medications.

Headaches are common in pregnancy and occur in women who do not usually suffer them. These may result from the increased blood supply to the head, or tension. You may find that overheated houses, offices, or stuffy atmospheres make you feel headachy and claustrophobic. If so, it is preferable to open windows or disappear outside for a breath of air, than to treat yourself with analgesics. If you must rid yourself of the pain of a headache, take Tylenol rather than aspirin. If headaches persist, see your doctor. If you are a migraine sufferer, you may not use preparations containing ergot. You will have to rely on other analgesics.

Varicose veins are quite likely to increase, especially if this is your second or third pregnancy. Some women are genetically predisposed to varicose veins. Pregnancy aggravates them and causes more to appear. There is little that can be done to prevent this. Avoid excessive weight gain and too much stand-ing still. If you are standing at the stove, or in the office or factory, for example, always take little steps and go up and down on your toes, as the calf muscles are strong pumps and will stop the blood from accumulating in the veins. You can also elevate your bed by placing bricks under the front of it to encourage venous return at night. Your doctor may prescribe support hose, which will keep the veins collapsed and encourage venous re-turn. Remember, such hose must be worn all day; it will not help just to wear them for a couple of hours at a time. Varicose veins must never be operated on or injected during pregnancy. The need for surgery must be reassessed 6 months after the birth, when the effects of the pregnancy will have disappeared. Varicose veins may also develop in the vulva, but little can be done other than to rest.

Heartburn is an occupational hazard of pregnancy. You should avoid greasy foods, or any food that seems to aggravate the condition. Gelusil or Maalox can be used in moderation to re-lieve symptoms.

Frequent urination is also extremely common, sometimes making life very difficult if you are out for a full day and do not know where to find a toilet. Try to regulate fluid intake till this symptom diminishes. Also, empty your bladder as soon as the urge occurs and do not let it overfill. Avoid too much coffee and tea, as these have a pronounced diuretic effect on some people. If your urine starts to burn, it may mean infection, so see your doctor.

Hemorrhoids: These are varicose veins in the anal canal, and they are common during pregnancy and especially if you have varicose veins of the legs. Try to avoid becoming constipated, as straining to evacuate the bowel can aggravate the hemor-rhoids. For itching or bleeding, you can use Anusol supposito-ries. As hemorrhoids usually shrink after birth, surgical treatment or injection treatments should be delayed until some months after pregnancy.

Abdominal (stomach) pain: The enlarging uterus may cause different uncomfortable sensations in the abdomen.

Heaviness may be experienced owing to the pressure of the uterus, and this is best dealt with by lying on one's back or side.

Pain in either side of the lower abdomen may be due to stretching of the cordlike ligaments (round ligaments) that support the uterus, very much like the supports of a tent. The tender structures can be rolled under the hand. Treatment is by resting on the side with legs curled, and local heat and pain relievers.

Appendicitis is rare in pregnancy.

Swelling (edema): Swelling of the feet and ankles is common in late pregnancy, especially in the summer. It is best treated by elevation of the legs to improve the circulation. Diuretics must not be used in pregnancy. Swelling of the rest of the body (face, hands) must be reported to your doctor, as it may indicate pre-eclampsia.

Danger signals

When should you contact your doctor in early pregnancy?

The answer is whenever you are concerned or have a question. However, here are some signs to watch out for.

Bleeding—any bleeding must be reported. This includes a brown discharge, as well as any flow of blood.

Low abdominal cramps or pain increasing in severity over a time, as this may indicate premature labor or miscarriage.

Swelling of the hands or feet, headache, blurring of vision.

General medical symptoms such as a fever.

Tender lesions of the labia that might be herpes.

Vaginal discharges that irritate.

Contact with or suspicion of German measles (rubella), hepatitis.

DRUGS: MEDICAL AND SOCIAL

If you are wondering what drugs or medications are safe to use in pregnancy, remember just one point: basically all agents cross the placenta and may affect the baby directly or, secondarily, affect you. Do not take anything unless specifically prescribed by your doctor (and then only if the drug has been checked in the latest medical reference as to its safety in pregnancy). As you will have discovered from the first chapter, the primary danger period for the use of any drugs or medication is the first 10 to 12 weeks of fetal life (14 weeks of traditional pregnancy dating) or the whole of the first trimester. Any inadvertent use of a harmful self-prescribed over-the-counter medication or a social drug might ruin your baby's chance of a normal life before life has really begun.

Sleeping pills: Most women find the first trimester the best cure for insomnia ever invented! But if you really need something to help you sleep, then the occasional use of phenobarbital will be the safest remedy. The medication may put your baby to sleep as well as you. But it will not cause any fetal abnormalities or harm. Do not take anything you have seen advertised without asking your doctor.

Tranquilizers: You may find yourself weepy and emotional in the early part of pregnancy, a time when the hormonal changes can leave you feeling depressed. Some patients on their third or fourth pregnancy, with young children at home, feel so tired and unable to cope they beg for tranquilizers to see them through.

Diazepam (Valium) and chlordiazepoxide (Librium) used to be prescribed quite regularly to women in labor as sedatives, but now there are suspicions of their link with birth defects, so I advise against them at any time of pregnancy. In fact, the use of any tranquilizers is now contraindicated, even including meprobamate (Equanil, Miltown).

If you were taking Valium before realizing you were pregnant, speak to your doctor about it, but do not panic. The work linking it to birth defects (of the palate) is not conclusive, and it would probably not be a reason for terminating a pregnancy.

Lithium, which is used to treat certain depressive disorders, is being implicated as a major cause of birth defects, and figures not yet published indicate that 10 percent of women who take lithium will give birth to a child with some defect.

Any antidepressants of the tricyclic group (monoamine oxidase inhibitors) should be avoided in pregnancy as they, too, have been associated with birth defects. Your doctor must be told if you are, or have been, using them. It is advisable for women on antidepressants to discuss pregnancy with their doctors *before* conceiving. Even if you are depressed by your marriage, relationship, or because of an unwanted pregnancy, do not turn to antidepressants. Instead, seek the support of your doctor or of a friend or relative if your husband is not available or sympathetic. It will be better to endure the emotional strain now (it should pass by the time you enter the second trimester), than to burden yourself with guilt and with the emotional, physical, and financial strain if your baby is born with a birth defect.

Over-the-counter medications: Aspirin should not be taken during pregnancy, as it has been associated with minor birth defects (see page 31). High-dose vitaminds are to be avoided unless they are vitamins for pregnant women prescribed by your doctor (see page 127).

SEX AND YOUR EMOTIONS

Is sex safe in pregnancy?

Let me clear up the most prevalent myth about sex and pregnancy. Intercourse itself will not harm your baby, nor will it lead to an early miscarriage. Despite controversial reports to the contrary, it is generally accepted that as long as you do not fall into one of the high-risk categories (see below), any version of sexual intercourse and other forms of sexual activity are safe throughout the whole of your pregnancy.

I believe that sexual activity between husband and wife is important during pregnancy to ensure that neither partner loses touch with the source of this intimate and potentially erotic thing that has happened to you both—a baby! The pregnant woman should remember that while she is enjoying all the physiological changes and spiritual enlargements of the developing relationship between fetus and self, her husband is very much an outsider. He helped start the whole thing off, but has been left on the base line to look and observe. You can help him feel involved by allowing him intimacy with your body, letting him touch, feel the movements of the fetus and the linear contours himself.

First, though, I should elaborate on who might be in the high-risk categories advised to abstain from full intercourse for certain periods of the pregnancy. If you have a history of sponteous miscarriages, penetration and ejaculation into the vagina should be avoided until you are beyond the point of your previous miscarriage by some weeks. The reason intercourse might stimulate miscarriage is not clear, but it could be a mechanical result of the penis pressing against the cervix. It is more likely that the content of prostaglandin in seminal fluid induces abortion. (On pages 19–20 there is a discussion of the use of prostaglandins in bringing on early therapeutic abortions.) Prostaglandin is found throughout our bodies but has a particularly high concentration in male semen and, if applied to the cervix or into the vagina, may cause uterine contractions. Whether the prostaglandin in male ejaculate is sufficient to trigger an early abortion is not really known, but there may be danger if you are prone to abortions.

Intercourse is also discouraged if you have been in premature labor (labor before 36 weeks), have any bleeding during pregnancy, or if your cervix is dilated—which your doctor will be able to tell from the internal examination in late pregnancy. If the membranes are showing, they run a greater risk of becoming infected or they can rupture and allow penetration of bacteria into the uterus.

What about deep penetration and orgasm?

It would be easy to disparage fears that deep penetration in intercourse will set off a miscarriage. But I do believe there is an ancient taboo in all of us, almost like the taboo against incest, that makes pregnant women fear aggressive penetrating sex. In fact, there is nothing to suggest that the deeper the penile penetration the more vulnerable you are to miscarriage. In the third trimester, you have to be careful not to allow too deep penetration. But in early pregnancy there is really nothing to fear, providing you have experienced no danger signals.

Orgasm, which has been shown to cause uterine contractions, also frightens some pregnant women who feel the contractions will encourage premature labor or miscarriage. But your body will only miscarry or go into premature labor if the hormonal support system of the pregnancy fails to operate. The orgasmic contractions you experience will not fool your uterus into thinking its time to end the pregnancy!

You and your husband can continue to enjoy sexual activity without any fear or guilt. You may notice, however, an alteration in your experience of orgasm. Many women say that they do not get the same tension release from orgasm during pregnancy as in the nonpregnant state. It is quite likely that this is due to the engorgement of the genital area with extra blood. Although the intensity of your orgasms may diminish, you are likely to discover that you find increased pleasure in foreplay, stroking, caressing, being loved, and showing love. Whatever your experience, it will last only as long as the pregnancy and does not mean your sex life is ruined, or improved, forever.

If you do not feel like sex, does it mean there is something wrong with your marriage?

Having explained that intercourse is safe for the sexually interested, I must also make it clear that many women lose much of their libido during the first trimester of pregnancy. This is actually a physiological response of pregnancy, owing to the hormonal changes. It is normal and not something to worry about. It does not mean your relationship with your husband is over, or irrevocably changed. In fact, within a few weeks, in the middle trimester, your libido will probably come back as never before. You will most likely enter a phase of well-being and rosy health; feeling sensual, loved, and extremely contented with the pregnancy.

There are other reasons a woman may lose interest in sex in the first trimester. First, there may be the problem of nausea or vomiting. Your taste buds in the first trimester feel off-center; your sense of smell has changed, and you probably are not picking up on the scents and aromas that would normally lead you to arousal. Feeling nauseated also means your mouth does not salivate with pleasure. All you may want to do is fall asleep and forget how rotten you are feeling.

Sleepiness and fatigue associated with the first trimester are also good antiaphrodisiacs. How can you work up the energy for prolonged sessions of lovemaking when you can hardly stagger from the sofa to the bed? A pregnant woman already coping with the strains of caring for a toddler may feel particularly fatigued.

It is of course advisable to talk over any temporary sexual problems with your husband to prevent his feeling jealous of the baby's place in your life, or that he has been made into an outcast. Most men are sensitive to their wives' changed feelings in early pregnancy, particularly if they understand that those feelings should improve within a few weeks. If *you* need to read books to explain the mysteries of pregnancy to you, do not expect your husband miraculously to accept and understand. Try to explain what is happening to you as you go along.

There is an area of your feelings, however, that you may find hard to discuss with him. Many women describe the feeling of being invaded by their husbands, particularly in the first trimester. A usually loving wife cannot bear to feel her husband's arms around her. She does not want her breasts caressed, since it makes them feel more tender. She resents having to give in to his need for sexual pleasure when she has her own changing body to come to terms with. She does not want him to interrupt the sensitive and slowly developing relationship between herself and the baby.

If you are feeling anything along those lines, rather than worrying unduly, you should assume that the hostility will pass as you enter the second and third trimesters. By then you will be feeling more confident of the safety of your pregnancy. You will have a belly to show to the world.

Try to bring your husband into the picture by describing some of what you feel. Hopefully, he will love you all the more for it and will feel protective rather than antagonistic to you in this sometimes difficult period.

Moving into the second trimester usually means you leave behind the negative, rather inward-looking feelings, and turn to a more exciting, decidedly positive attitude toward the pregnancy and future.

Can you have oral sex?

You may continue to practice oral sex during pregnancy. As prostaglandins (in seminal fluid) are absorbed through the membranes of the mouth it is probably a good idea to abstain from this practice early in pregnancy if you have a history of miscarriages, or in late pregnancy if you have been in premature labor.

Cunnilingus may be continued in pregnancy if this is your practice. However, your husband must not blow into your vagina, since, in pregnancy, there are so many extra blood vessels in that region that there is a very real risk of an air embolism, which can be very dangerous for you. If your husband has fever blisters on his mouth or herpes in the mouth, cunnilingus is contraindicated.

Can anal intercourse be continued in pregnancy?

You may continue to practice anal intercourse unless your doctor has forbidden vaginal intercourse because of the risk of spontaneous abortion. Then you must not practice anal penetration either, as the penis can hit up against the back of the uterus, and there is the same risk of introducing bacteria into the cervix and uterus. If anal penetration by the penis is followed by any form of vaginal penetration, it could also introduce an excessive amount of bacteria into the vagina that could further increase the risk of infection.

Are there any sexual positions that might be harmful?

Any position is fine for sexual activity. In the first trimester, there is nothing to prevent you from enjoying the man-on-top position. His weight is not going to affect the abdomen, and you will not find it uncomfortable. If rear entry or woman-on-top are more comfortable for you with a large belly, there is no danger in such positions. Essentially you do not have to change your sexual practices in pregnancy. If certain aspects bother you, then discuss these with your obstetrician.

Masturbation is safe in pregnancy. However, be careful of substances introduced into the vagina. You do not want to use any medicated creams that might be absorbed into the bloodstream. Vibrators are less safe during pregnancy, and should not be used to penetrate the vagina. There should be no harm if one is used just to stimulate the clitoris.

Can you douche?

You do not need to douche in pregnancy (unless your doctor has advised it as a treatment for Trichomonas). The acidy white discharge that may be slightly discomforting or embarrassing to you is a normal condition of pregnancy. It is in fact helping to prevent infection by keeping bacteria from passing into the pelvis. Because of this preventive feature, the discharge should not be eradicated. I suggest, therefore, that you do not douche while pregnant, as you will be tampering with the body's own natural chemical balance created specifically for the pregnant state.

Douching in itself—introducing liquid into the vagina—will not harm the baby. If one is compelled to douche, plain water or a combination of vinegar and water is recommended. However, the commonly used Betadine douche has been shown to cause raised levels of iodine in the amniotic fluid, which may affect the baby's developing thyroid. My advice is to avoid this brand and probably other douches containing deodorizing chemicals. Douching is seldom necessary in pregnancy.

Can depression or a major argument affect a pregnancy?

If your due date is near, there is a chance that severe mental stress, particularly shock or fright, can precipitate the onset of early labor possibly owing to an increase of adrenaline in your system. If contractions should begin, however, it is very likely that they will subside once you have been investigated, and made to rest, and your pregnancy will return to normal.

Obviously the ideal situation for pregnancy is one in which you are happy to be pregnant and involved in a good loving relationship with your husband. But it is not always possible to arrange life like that. Do be reassured, however, if you are going through a period of great emotional stress that it will not in itself harm the baby. I had a patient who discovered halfway through her first pregnancy that her husband was having an affair with a younger woman and that he wanted to leave her. When she learned what was happening, my patient was so distraught that her weight suddenly dropped, her blood pressure rose, and we hospitalized her once or twice before the onset of labor. Each time she was in the hospital the worries abated, and the pregnancy finally came to term in a normal fashion. The baby was born at a good weight and very healthy. I really did appreciate the strain this woman was under, but her husband's disaffection only seemed to strengthen her need to have the baby. She was determined that her own emotional reactions were not going to hinder her child's well-being.

It is a good general rule to try to keep calm at work, and put extra effort into your relationship at home. If this is a first pregnancy, remember that your husband is undergoing a lot of emotional stress, too, wondering about what is going to happen to your life together once you are parents, what this pregnancy means to him, and the amount of financial and emotional commitment he is suddenly pledged to. If he is undergoing pressure at work on top of all this, it may become overwhelming. If he does become irritable or argumentative, do try to be sympathetic and listen to his woes. I do not mean to be antifeminist by taking "his" side, but he may well feel you have everything going for you, with the baby tucked there under your belt, while he has nothing—not even you. Be positive in your love, and if he should start an argument, rather than let him provoke you to anger or overexcitement, remain calm and reassuring.

Don't forget that your fears and negative feelings may be there just below the surface too. Many women planning to go back to work once they have had the baby become extremely worried about finding a baby-sitter or day care, whether they will be able to leave the baby with a stranger; they worry about losing their friends and changing their life style; they worry about losing their husband to another woman. Many women experience strong negative feelings about the pregnancy in the first trimester. It was all a dreadful mistake! They do not really want to be mothers! They have always been young and single, and how are they going to change into this responsive, all-caring, all-curing mythical figure they call Mom? One of my patients made me laugh the other day when she went into a labor a few weeks early. I informed her she would be having her baby that same night. "Is it too late for an abortion?" she ruefully asked. Later she confessed that, there in my office, it had flashed upon her in a revelation that the pregnancy had been a game. She had enjoyed playing "mother-to-be," putting on the big clothes, watching her belly grow, but she had never really imagined herself with a *baby*.

You need have no fear that your not-quite-what-the-doctor-ordered emotional responses will be felt by the baby. He or she is quite happy swimming in the amniotic sac, oblivious to your confusions. You will probably have flashes of negative feelings throughout your parenthood. Few parents are untouched this way.

Most women who come to an obstetrician for their first pregnancy are nervous about having a baby. Some are terrified of pain and feel they will fail at natural childbirth; others fear miscarriage, stillbirth, or giving birth to a baby with some defect.

But these feelings will not affect the pregnancy in actuality. And you might be reassured to know that most women experience one or more of these confusing feelings.

EXERCISE AND TRAVEL

Generally speaking, my attitude to exercise in pregnancy is that as long as you are healthy and everything proceeds normally with the pregnancy, then you can exercise to any degree that feels comfortable. You can look back to pages 50–55 for an extended discussion on the relative virtues and disadvantages of certain types of exercise, the sports that are contraindicated, and on the philosophy of sport in pregnancy today.

Travel

In the first trimester, you will not notice any discomfort from a long journey other than the natural discomforts caused by nausea, vomiting, or sleepiness. Do not take drugs to ease air-sickness. It is unlikely you will feel any more nauseated than usual on board a plane, and preventive medications might harm the baby. Do not drink alcohol to soothe your nerves either. The danger of any drugs will far outweigh the extent of your own discomfort or anxiety, which will be short-lived.

If you are planning a journey and have time to make advance arrangements, I strongly advise you to wait until the second trimester. During those 3 months, you will feel at your fittest and best in the pregnancy. You will have the most stamina for enduring long hours of sitting in cramped positions. If you are going to be away for longer than 4 weeks, you should discuss this with your obstetrician, as he or she may want you to check in with a colleague in the town or country you are visiting. Or failing that, it might be advisable to take along a copy of the doctor's notes on the pregnancy so far, should you need to visit another doctor.

Airline travel should be perfectly all right as long as the flight is with a major commercial company, as all their vessels are pressurized. If you are flying in a small unpressurized plane, you should not go above 8,000 feet because the decrease in oxygen might harm the baby. Airlines have no official policy against air travel in the early months of pregnancy.

If you have previously miscarried or showed any indications of miscarrying, then I would advise against air travel, since, if anything begins to go wrong, there is no way of helping you once you are on a long flight to a distant place.

Should you be vaccinated before travel?

Before planning travel to some far-off country, it is very important that you be aware of the latest rulings on vaccinations during pregnancy. If you know you are pregnant, or could be, you must refuse to have the following vaccinations for fear they could harm the baby.

You *cannot* be vaccinated against:

Smallpox or Typhoid Fever—unless you have been exposed, or are in an epidemic. Even then the bad effects of the live vaccine will have to be weighed against the risks to the baby.

Yellow Fever—unless there has been direct exposure.

You *may* be vaccinated against:

Cholera—the vaccine is probably not harmful, and you may need it to satisfy travel requirements to Southeast Asia.

Rabies and Tetanus—if there is any indication of exposure.

Malaria—Chloroquine may be used but *only* if you are going to an endemic area.

Polio vaccine may be administered in pregnancy if the patient is not already immune.

Can you go through the X-ray machines at airports?

Many women express their fears of the X-ray machines used in security checks at airports. The FAA security department points out that you do not go through the X-ray machine yourself, but through the metal detector, which does not emit radiation and which has been proved safe even for cardiac patients wearing pacemakers. Your baggage goes through the X-ray machine, which emits a very low amount of background radiation. These machines have been proved harmless even to photographic film. As the FAA points out, security personnel wear radiation-detecting badges, and pregnant women are not precluded from working by the X-ray machines or the metal detectors. No badge has so far, in all the years they have been used, shown any trace of radioactivity. The official view, therefore, is that the machines are quite safe. My own view is that if you wish to minimize the level of any radiation to which you are exposed during pregnancy, you should let your husband handle the luggage and try to walk away from the X-ray machine. You may request a physical check if you wish. But for that you will have to go to a private room and wait until a member of the security staff is available.

WORK

Should you cut down on your working hours in early pregnancy?

It would actually make good sense to insist pregnant women took the *first* 3 months off work, rather than the last 3. In the first trimester many women find it is an uphill battle to keep up with the job because of nausea and sleepiness. Do not expect miracles of yourself. You will probably not work as well during this period as in your nonpregnant state. I know that many women do not tell their boss or employer about the pregnancy until they are beginning to "show." However, remember that if you do not let anyone know, you cannot expect sympathy for poor work in the first trimester.

During these first 3 months, try to arrange a 4-day week, or to be allowed to go home earlier in the afternoons than usual. If you find the courage to break the news now to your boss, you will have a chance to explain that this tiredness will not last. It should disappear by the time you are 12 to 14 weeks pregnant and then you should find renewed vigor and energy. Try to encourage your boss's emotional support (and it is not only male bosses who often prove hostile to a pregnant worker or colleague).

CHAPTER
3
The Second Trimester
14–28 WEEKS

Once in the second trimester you are well on the way in the pregnancy. Your mind will be more at ease, and a new sense of self-confidence and assurance should replace the fatigue and sometimes negative feelings of the past 3 months. Some of the ease will come from physiological changes, for the time that you might have miscarried on a hormonal basis has now passed and you can be free of that fear. At about 10 to 12 weeks the luteo-placental shift occurs as the hormonal support system shifts from the corpus luteum to the placenta, which is now responsible for hormone production (see page 9). You now have a fetus in the uterus, no longer an embryo. Although the fetus is not yet capable of independent life, all its major organs have developed and it will continue to gain in size, weight, and maturity.

What changes can you expect in yourself?

With the baby's increased size, nervous system, and muscular development it begins to move about more in the amniotic sac and, any time between 18 to 22 weeks, you will feel its first movements, known as quickening.

The position of the baby at this stage varies because of the relatively large amount of amniotic fluid compared to the small size of the fetus. The baby can move around, swim up and down, and may be in any position on any particular day. It is immaterial which way the baby lies right now and your doctor will not begin to check for fetal position until the twenty-fourth week.

Among the other changes you should notice will be a mood change. As the nausea and vomiting disappear between the twelfth and the sixteenth week (in most pregnancies), your energy and sense of fun will return, as will your libido. The nipples will also begin to secrete colostrum. Pigmentation about the abdomen and face may increase. You should be careful about urinary infections now, because the ureters get compressed by the uterus as it lifts from the pelvis into the abdomen and displaces the bowel. Once the uterus is up from the pelvis your waistline will begin to disappear and you will begin to wear maternity clothes. All of which will help you be more positive about the pregnancy.

Besides routine prenatal care at this stage, your doctor will be concentrating on measuring the adequate growth of the fetus. Toward the end of this trimester any inadequacy in the baby's nutrition or oxygen (intrauterine growth retardation or IUGR) will begin to show in your low weight gain, which is one reason your weight will be checked at each office visit.

What changes are happening to the baby?

Twelfth week after conception (which compares to the fourteenth week of traditional pregnancy dating): Bodily changes are evident in the fetus. The neck has lengthened, and its head is not so bent on the chest. The abdominal wall closes, concealing the intestines, which until then have been on the outside.

Fourteenth week after conception: All the baby's joints are moving, fingernails and toenails are grown. A fine hair called lanugo covers the whole of its body. The baby is also covered with a greasy substance called vernix, which protects its skin from the watery environment. The baby is 16 centimeters (6¼ inches) long and weighs 35 grams (1¼ ounces).

Eighteenth week after conception: The baby is growing rapidly both in length and weight. It has hair on its head and, because of its increased muscle development, it makes some very active movements that can be felt by the mother. There is still a relatively large amount of amniotic fluid in which the baby swims. It is about 25½ centimeters (10 inches) long, and weighs around 340 grams (nearly 12 ounces).

Twenty-second week after conception: The baby is now about 35½ centimeters (14 inches) long and weighs around 570 grams (1¼ pounds).

Twenty-sixth week after conception: The baby's head is only slightly larger in proportion to its body. It should be about 37 centimeters (14½ inches) long, and will weigh 900 grams (nearly 2 pounds).

The fetus is now regarded as viable, that is, capable of independent life. Any birth from this point on is called premature, whereas before this time it would have been called a miscarriage. Legally, if the baby is born, it must be registered, and if it dies, it must be buried. With modern neonatal care any baby born from here on in has almost a 70 percent chance of survival, provided there are no congenital abnormalities or injuries at birth. The percentage varies, depending on the type of hospital where the baby is delivered. The intensive care neonatal units are only found in major teaching hospitals.

THE MOTHER'S HEALTH AND CONDITION

If you do not feel quickening, does it mean something is wrong?

The first fetal movements, known as quickening, are usually felt at some time between 18 and 22 weeks. The word quickening has an almost biblical ring, and the sensation is not anything definite or scientific; you will experience it as a feeling that something moved inside you, rather like a stomach rumble. Some women describe it as a pulsation, a flutter, or as a hollow feeling inside. If you do not feel quickening at what you consider to be the right time, do not worry. Often in a first pregnancy the movements are felt later. If your doctor is satisfied with the pregnancy and can hear the heartbeats with the Fetone at your regular visits, then you need have no concern. If too much time passes and you still report not feeling movements, your doctor might investigate by ultrasound as there is a small possibility of an anterior placenta muffling the sensations. Again that would not be cause for concern, though it is wise for your doctor to know about it as soon as possible.

Once you do begin to feel the fetal movements, you should have some sensation every day. If you do not feel them for more than 12 hours, do tell your doctor. This is a very unusual time for the baby just to die inside you, but you should be investigated to see that all is well if movements cease. (For more information on fetal movements, see pages 227–231.)

If you look small, is it a bad sign?

Your weight will continue to rise because, as you can see from the previous pages, the baby's weight is increasing rapidly, and this will show up on your scale. But the second trimester is a classic time for women to be told they look "small." Your size will depend on many factors, such as your build, stature (tall women tend to hide pregnancy better at this stage), and carriage. It also depends on the amount of amniotic fluid you are carrying. If your doctor is satisfied with the progress of the pregnancy, so should you be. Your size will have nothing to do with the well-being of the baby. You will get big enough in time.

If you start to feel contractions, is this a danger sign?

Many women are nervous when they first feel tightenings of the uterus which are called Braxton Hicks contractions (named after the obstetrician who first discovered their purpose in pregnancy). These mild uterine contractions, in fact, happen throughout your life and not only in pregnancy. Other parts of the body also contract and relax regularly throughout life—such as the heart, intestines, and blood vessels. In pregnancy, the enlarged uterus makes you aware of the contractions, usually some time after the twentieth week.

Braxton Hicks contractions can be regarded as a trial run for labor, though really they are organizing the smooth running of the whole pregnancy. Their effect is to squeeze out the blood from the uterine veins, leaving them to be refilled with fresh blood. They encourage the baby to move about and force it to use its muscles. They help to stretch out the lower part of the uterus, preparing it for labor.

How do you know they are Braxton Hicks contractions and not labor pains? Actually, Braxton Hicks may sometimes be uncomfortable but they are never increasingly so. They are noticed as a hardening of the uterus, which lasts for 20 to 30 seconds and seldom occur any more frequently than once every 15 to 20 minutes. They do not become more frequent over a period of hours. There is never any loss of blood at the same time, whereas the onset of labor is often accompanied by a show of blood and mucus.

What will the doctor be checking for during your visits?

Regular visits in the second trimester are usually every 4 weeks from the fourteenth to the thirty-second week (after which they become more frequent). This is generally a calm time for doctor and patient, who are not overburdened with worries or anxieties; but the doctor will be making sure that everything progresses normally.

Your doctor may do a second blood count toward the end of this trimester if you were anemic, and retest for antibodies if you are Rh negative. Ultrasound (see pages 192–193) may be performed to check the maturity of the baby. Otherwise, your blood pressure and urine will be checked, you will hear the baby's heartbeat, and you will be weighed. Internal examinations are not usually done at this time.

The doctor or nurse will talk to you about prenatal classes, and about your preference for any particular style of delivery, such as Lamaze, Leboyer, or Bradley. It is a good idea to attend prenatal classes, as you will have more time for discussion about pregnancy and labor. As these classes are usually held in the evening, it gives your husband a chance to become more involved. Futher, you will meet other couples and you won't feel so alone.

Incompetent cervix: The condition reveals itself during this trimester, if it is going to occur. You need not worry unduly if your doctor discovers that your cervix is incompetent. It does not mean you are going to lose the baby. Your cervix should be long and tightly closed right now, but it may shorten and begin to open rather early, in which case treatment may be indicated. This condition is not common, but if you have regular contractions, any vaginal bleeding, or passage of mucus, these could be indications of an incompetent cervix and should be reported to your doctor.

The weakness of the cervix may have been caused by a previous induced abortion, especially if the pregnancy was advanced. It may also occur because of a congenital abnormality of your uterus. If you have had a previous second-trimester miscarriage, your doctor will also be on the lookout for premature opening of the cervix. Very often the cause of the cervical incompetence is not found.

The treatment for the condition is hospitalization and, after some bed rest, a suture or stitch will be placed in the cervix under general anesthesia. This is commonly called a Shirodkar suture. Your physical activity will be curtailed and you will be allowed no sexual intercourse for the rest of the pregnancy. The stitch is removed from the cervix once the baby is mature enough to be born, usually between 38 and 40 weeks of pregnancy. A general anesthetic or a regional anesthetic such as an epidural will be needed for placing the stitch, but not for its removal.

Pre-eclampsic toxemia: Another sign to be watched for in the middle trimester is a rise in blood pressure. One cause for a rise at this time is pre-eclampsia, a condition peculiar to pregnancy, which usually begins to show up at the end of the second trimester. With this condition, high blood pressure may be associated with swelling of the hands and feet, and there may be protein in the urine.

Pre-eclampsia used to be very serious, harming the baby and sometimes leading to convulsions in the mother. But now that good prenatal care is common, including the constant monitoring of blood pressure for any elevation, of urine for signs of protein, and of weight for fluid retention, this condition is not allowed to become severe. If it is detected, its seriousness can be minimized. Treatment of pre-eclampsia is by bed rest, occasionally a mild sedative, and a short spell of hospitalization. But it varies depending on its severity. You will be encouraged to give up work and to take it easy for the rest of the pregnancy, both emotionally and physically. You will also be seen more frequently by your obstetrician.

Baby as patient: Between 13 and 26 weeks the baby does

not need any particular treatment other than your good diet and supplemental vitamins prescribed by your obstetrician. If intrauterine growth retardation (IUGR) should occur, it can be detected by the end of the second trimester. The treatment would be bed rest, and you probably will be encouraged to give up work. The second trimester is not ordinarily the stage, however, when special tests are done to measure fetal well-being—these are done in the third trimester. However, if yours is a high-risk pregnancy, or if there are other indications that such tests might be necessary, your doctor can investigate the health of the baby.

THE SECOND-TRIMESTER TESTS

Who is likely to be tested and by what sort of tests?

Having said that the second trimester is a calm time for both mother and doctor, one of waiting for the pregnancy to develop and for the fetus to grow, I do not want to overlook that to some women this is the time that tests may be done to tell her whether the fetus she is carrying is healthy and normal.

Any woman who is over thirty-five at the time of this pregnancy or who will be thirty-five when she has the baby, will have been waiting since her first booking visit for an *amniocentesis*. I doubt very much that your doctor will spring it on you by surprise, as the indications for amniocentesis will have been discussed much earlier in the pregnancy. I will explain amniocentesis and *ultrasound* fully in the following sections. There is also a newer test, still at research level, known as *fetoscopy*, which we may be hearing more of in the next few years.

Who will have an amniocentesis?

If you are reading ahead of your time in this chapter and are wondering why your doctor has not mentioned amniocentesis to you, let me describe the relatively small groups of women who fall into the high-risk categories indicating the beneficial value of amniocentesis.

Advanced parental age: The largest group of mothers presenting for amniocentesis are those of advanced maternal age. Pregnancy books that were written more than 3 to 5 years ago usually state that only pregnant women of forty or older are tested. But these days, as demand is so high, and as the results of the screening for Down's syndrome (Mongoloid) babies have been so successful, most major hospitals and genetics laboratories will test any pregnant woman of thirty-five or older (see page 83).

The presence of Down's syndrome is an important condition that we are able to diagnose from tests on amniotic fluid. Fetal cells are taken from the sample of fluid, they are grown, and the fetal chromosomes are studied and the condition can be diagnosed.

For a long time doctors have been able to associate this condition with advanced parental age and, as the numbers of older parents in America increase each year, amniocentesis (with the option to terminate the pregnancy if Down's syndrome is discovered) has been of great benefit to such parents. It has taken away the stigma attached to being "older" parents and the consequent fear that they are going to be punished with an abnormal baby for daring to start a family so late in life. Indeed, the trend toward having babies later in life continues to increase as women discover the virtues of concentrating on a career first and family later. The latest government projections on births associated with age show that by 1982 there will have been 138,418 births to women between the ages of thirty-five and thirty-nine. That is an increase of nearly 50 percent over the past 10 years. And by 1988, it is predicted that as many as 2,500 babies will be born to women over forty-four. Such figures show a great rise in the confidence and expectations of women planning to become mothers after the "traditional" age.

Doctors are aware of the changing life patterns of women today and I do hope that none of you find yourself looked down upon, or even laughed at, for becoming mothers after the first gray hairs have started to show!

Repeat spontaneous aborters: Anyone who has had three or more consecutive spontaneous miscarriages in previous consecutive pregnancies (see pages 77–78) is likely to have an amniocentesis, for a cause of these miscarriages is chromosomal abnormalities that have made previous conceptions incompatible with life. Your obstetrician will want to check, therefore, that this pregnancy you have carried to midterm is not affected by a similar defect. Middle-trimester amniocentesis is a great reassurance to such women.

Anyone who has previously given birth to a defective baby: If you have had the misfortune to give birth to a baby with, for example, anencephaly or spina bifida (in which cases the baby may have died within hours or days of birth); to a child with a sex-linked disorder such as hemophilia or Duchene muscular dystrophy (in such cases it might be advantageous to learn the sex of the baby, as a girl child would be free of the disorder); or to a previous Down's syndrome child, you would require amniocentesis during your next pregnancy.

Tay-Sachs carriers: If your husband is a carrier of the Tay-Sachs disease and you were already pregnant when this was discovered, you would have to have amniocentesis to find out if your baby has the disease (see page 177). Recently a test on the pregnant mother's blood has been developed as well, and this may avoid having to have an amniocentesis.

History of congenital abnormality: If there is a history of a congenital abnormality in your family, in your husband's family, or in a child born to you from a previous marriage, you may need an amniocentesis, which should help put your mind at rest during this pregnancy.

Close kinship: If you and your husband are first cousins, even without a recent family history of congenital abnormalities, the risks of your producing a child with a genetic defect are greatly increased (see pages 79–80).

Fertility drugs: If you were taking a fertility drug such as Pergonal or Clomid before getting pregnant, you should discuss amniocentesis with your obstetrician as there is a slightly higher risk to your baby of a birth defect.

Exactly what does amniocentesis discover about the baby?

One unfortunate misconception about amniocentesis, is the belief that once the results are received and the news is good, it *guarantees* a baby will be born without any defect. However, this is not always true. Amniocentesis is basically a test on the chromosomes that can detect a chromosomal abnormality in the fetus. Tests are also done on the baby's biochemical makeup and so certain results are available on disorders that are chemical in nature. In the next section, to make this clear, I will explain what does *not* show up through amniocentesis. For now, let me explain further about the disorders that are distinguished by amniotic fluid culture. For more information on chromosomal makeup and genetic disorders you might like to turn back to Chapter 1, pages 3–84, where the role of genetics counseling and screening for certain genetic diseases was discussed.

Genetics laboratories connected with teaching hospitals can do up to forty tests on the amniotic fluid sample taken from you during amniocentesis. But the only tests that you will probably find relevant are those for the more common disorders whose names have become familiar among prospective parents: Down's syndrome, neural tube defects (such as spina bifida, anencephaly, meningocele), and Tay-Sachs. One other determination that can be made through amniocentesis is usually of great interest—the sex of the child.

Down's syndrome: In the amniotic fluid are cells from the fetus that are washed off as the baby moves around in its

Risk of having a liveborn child with Down's syndrome by one year maternal age intervals from ages 20–49 years.

MATERNAL AGE	RISK OF DOWN'S SYNDROME
20	1/1923
21	1/1695
22	1/1538
23	1/1408
24	1/1299
25	1/1205
26	1/1124
27	1/1053
28	1/990
29	1/935
30	1/885
31	1/826
32	1/725
33	1/592
34	1/465
35	1/365
36	1/287
37	1/225
38	1/177
39	1/139
40	1/90
41	1/85
42	1/67
43	1/53
44	1/41
45	1/32
46	1/25
47	1/20
48	1/16
49	1/12

As you can see from the table, the risk of having a Down's syndrome baby changes appreciably from age 37. Many medical centers will now perform amniocentesis on women who are 35 years or over.

Data of Hook and Chambers (1977), from the World Symposium of Perinatal Medicine, San Francisco, 1981.

water cocoon. These cells are cultured on a slide much as yours would be if a blood sample had been taken from your arm to investigate your own chromosomal makeup (see page 162 on carrier screening for Down's syndrome).

The chances of producing a child with a chromosomal problem increase rapidly with the mother's advancing age. From age thirty to thirty-five the rise is gradual, but, after thirty-five, it becomes more dramatic—increasing from 1 in 800 to 1 in 400 births. If you are younger than thirty-five but have previously had a child with Down's syndrome, similar tests on the fetal cells will be done, as the recurrence rate is about 1 percent (four times higher than the average risk). (For an explanation of why Down's syndrome occurs, see pages 73–74.)

Spina bifida, anencephaly, or meningomyelocele: These disorders are collectively known as neural tube defects and they result from an accident during the formation of the baby's brain and spinal cord that, you may remember from Chapter 1 (pages 9–10), happens in the first 4 weeks of fetal life (that is, 4 weeks dating from conception). Neural tube defects are not genetically passed on. But if you have previously given birth to a baby with such a defect, there is a 1 in 20, or 5 percent, chance of your baby's having the disorder (or that you will miscarry because the fetus is abnormal) in *each* future pregnancy.

What is a neural tube defect? It sounds strange and does need some explanation. At about the fourth week of fetal life, a fault can occur in the baby's development: an opening in the skull or the spinal cord does not close and spinal fluid (which surrounds the brain and spinal cord) leaks into the amniotic fluid. Spinal fluid contains a large amount of a substance called alpha-fetoprotein (AFP). Normally there is only a small amount of this substance in amniotic fluid, although there is always some evidence of it. An elevated level of alpha-fetoprotein may indicate that the spinal fluid has been leaking into the amniotic fluid from an opening in the fetal skull or spine. However, because a raised level alone of AFP does not confirm a neural tube defect, your doctor will perform an ultrasound scan to support the finding. Sometimes an elevated AFP is a false positive reaction and is actually high for some other unrelated reason, and is not due to a neural tube defect.

Although women having amniocentesis because of their age will routinely have the AFP level measured, the opposite is not true. If your amniocentesis is performed primarily to investigate the AFP level, you will not routinely receive the chromosomal analysis for Down's syndrome, unless your doctor specifically requests it.

Tay-Sachs: As explained on page 163, amniocentesis will reveal if your baby is suffering from this disorder.

Sex of the child: One positive result for many prospective parents, and often the one they irrationally worry about most, is determining whether they are having a boy or a girl. When the amniocentesis results come through, you can find out whether your baby is the sex you secretly hoped for, or you can choose to wait until delivery as was usual in the past.

Why do you have to go for genetics counseling before amniocentesis?

One thing you must understand is that amniocentesis itself does not show up all genetic diseases. And although a wide variety of tests is available on the amniotic fluid culture, not all laboratories can do all of them. Tests for Down's syndrome have become standard, but those for rare disorders may be at a research level and not widely available. If your amniotic fluid is tested in New York, for example, and you are a candidate for a very rare disorder the test for which is only available in San Francisco, the fluid may have to be sent there (or anywhere around the world).

For example, the March of Dimes has a story about a child who had MMA (Methylmalonic Acidemia) *in utero.* MMA is a very rare enzyme deficiency resulting in mental retardation and early death. The mother previously had a child who was born with the disorder and died after a few weeks of life. In the second pregnancy, the mother was desperate to discover before the baby's birth whether it, too, had MMA. The genetics counselor advised that a sample of her amniotic fluid be sent to Yale, where research was being done on the disease. The result was almost tragic because the baby did have MMA. But this story had a happy ending because the research work at Yale had led them to an *in utero* treatment of the disease. While still in the uterus, the baby was treated by vitamin injections into the mother. An abnormal fetus became a normal baby by the miracle of research becoming available at the right time and in the right place. So sometimes when you are wondering why they have to do all these tests on your amniotic fluid, bear such stories in mind. Without constant research, no such new breakthroughs would ever occur.

Genetics laboratories accept couples for pre-amniocentesis counseling for the following reasons: if they are of advanced parental age; if they have previously given birth to a baby with a chromosomal abnormality; if they are known to be carriers of a chromosomal translocation or suffer from mosaicism; if they are carriers of such recessive genetic diseases as Tay-Sachs; if they are carriers of sex-linked disorders such as hemophilia or Duchene muscular dystrophy; if they have previously had a child with either spina bifida or anencephaly; if ultrasound or blood alpha-fetoprotein testing is abnormal; if their family histories include the birth of a child with a congenital abnormality.

Can you refuse genetics counseling?

This section is included because I am aware, despite my previous comments, that many women do not particularly like the counseling session. To some it may seem unnecessarily expensive if they are getting a result anyway, and when they have the worries of the doctor's and hospital bills to cover, it can appear burdensome. Also, people fear that it can be very searching, especially if you are not married and have to go alone when the sessions are geared toward the couple, or if you had artificial insemination from a donor (AID).

For women who decide to forego genetics counseling, I must explain, then, that amniocentesis can be done in a doctor's office or in a hospital, in the usual way, using ultrasound. The amniotic fluid when drawn will then be sent for analysis to a commercial laboratory rather than to a hospital genetics laboratory. The commercial laboratory will test for Down's syndrome and Tay-Sachs. This alternative, alpha-fetoprotein (a screen for defects of nervous tissue), is available only to patients who need amniocentesis owing to advanced parental age, history of a previous Down's child, or because the father is a Tay-Sachs carrier. The commercial laboratories do not perform all the known tests, and they offer no counseling interview or follow-up talk after the amniocentesis. But by comparison, commercial testing is less expensive and, to some, a less harrowing experience. You must appreciate that part of the work offered by the medical schools' genetics laboratories is provided on behalf of research that, as I have just described, will be for the benefit of future prenatal diagnosis. Who knows? That diagnosis might one day help a member of your own family.

What does amniocentesis not test for?

Amniocentesis does not promise you a perfect baby. If you have read the sections in Chapter 1 on genetics and the various screening tests available for genetically inherited diseases, you may wonder, for example, how they can test, once you are pregnant, for sickle-cell anemia or for Cooley's anemia (beta-thalassemia).

By asking that question, you have hit the main point of what amniocentesis is not equipped to do. It cannot test for these genetic conditions. Those inherited defects are still very much with us and, for the present, the only tools we have for controlling them are the use of major screening programs of couples *before* they have babies.

Taking sickle-cell anemia and Cooley's anemia as examples (see page 73), the only way we can test to see whether the fetus has such diseases is to have a blood sample or a skin biopsy of the baby itself while it is in the uterus. This very new research procedure, known as *fetoscopy* (see below, pages 189–191), is currently available in a few major hospitals. Neither sickle-cell anemia nor beta-thalassemia is detectable by ultrasound or chromosomal analysis on amniotic fluid, as you cannot *see* a blood condition. Parents already identified as carriers will have been warned by a genetics counselor of the risks involved in future pregnancies and informed of treatment or care for children born with these conditions. (As with all genetically inherited disorders, not all babies conceived will be affected, but there is a 1 in 4 chance in *each* pregnancy of the child's having the disorder, a 1 in 4 chance it will be totally free of it, and a 2 in 4 chance that it will be normal but a carrier of the same disorder.)

Amniocentesis cannot detect defects of the body structure such as harelip, cleft palate, clubfoot, congenital heart disease, hypospadias, congenital hip dislocation, or pyloric stenosis (an obstruction of the lower end of the stomach into the small intestine). Defects such as these are not caused by chromosomal or genetic defects but are a result of what we term *multifactorial* reasons.

The problem may in part be due to a disorder of genes, but it may also result from some environmental hazard present either at conception or during the pregnancy. I cannot say exactly what those environmental hazards might have been. Obviously they include chemical inhalation or radiation; or it might be that some essential vitamin or mineral was missing from the mother's diet (and/or it might be missing in the soil or the water in the mother's area). Little is known about the effects of such hazards, which is why much more research must still be done.

However, the structural defects that I have described above are usually visible on ultrasound, as the newer, more refined machines give such a detailed picture that you can even see the baby's eyelids. And, I firmly believe, we are not far away from ultrasound so sophisticated that a skilled sonographer will be capable of picking up most structural defects.

If you are under thirty-five, can you request amniocentesis?

Younger women patients sometimes ask whether they can have amniocentesis even though they are not of the "eligible" age. It is incredible to think that a term most of us could hardly pronounce, let alone spell, a few years ago is now almost a household word (among propsective parents, at least). Many women are beginning to feel that the procedure should be their right in pregnancy. If older mothers can find out about birth defects, why can't they?

The chances of a younger mother (and remember the term "younger" means under thirty-five, so it still covers the large majority of pregnancies) giving birth to a child with a birth defect are much less, and in fact most such women do not seem unduly anxious about the prospects. However, that self-confidence can disappear quickly if you happen to meet a mother, or hear about a woman in your neighborhood who, for example, at twenty-eight had a second child born with Down's syndrome. Then suddenly the doctor is left to answer the unanswerable. How do you know it won't happen to me?

Let me say this: If you are genuinely and deeply concerned about such an eventuality, do speak to your doctor about it, honestly and urgently. Your doctor must understand that the level of anxiety you are suffering is not good for the pregnancy (although it will not affect the fetus itself). Most hospital genetics laboratories say they cannot handle amniocentesis and counseling for women under thirty-five because they are over-burdened with patients in the "older" group as it is. Moreover, before you begin to panic, do remember that the indicated age for amniocentesis was only dropped within the last couple of years to thirty-five-plus from over forty. The statistics do not rise alarmingly until women reach forty. And indeed, many hospitals still only see women over thirty-seven for routine am-niocentesis.

Before you decide that amniocentesis will ease your fears, do understand there are risks to both mother and fetus involved (see page 181), and that amniocentesis itself will not promise a clean bill of health for your baby. It will reassure you that your baby is not suffering from chromosomal abnormality or from a neural tube defect.

If you are truly concerned, there is nothing to prevent you from requesting the procedure from your doctor. Unless the physician has a completely different philosophy from yours, he or she may agree to perform it on request. Incidentally, most obstetricians would refuse amniocentesis on the grounds that you wanted only to find out the sex of the child. Choice of sex is not an indication for amniocentesis or termination of preg-nancy.

Can you refuse to have amniocentesis?

There are women for whom an amniocentesis is an unac-ceptable idea. These women, even if over thirty-five, do not feel anxious about the possibility of carrying a Down's baby and resent the technological intervention into what should be the natural process of pregnancy. They may have had previous children and cannot believe it could happen to them, or they may be morally or religiously opposed to the termination of pregnancy—so even if the fetus were found to be abnormal it would not alter their decision on carrying it to term.

The simple answer is, of course you can refuse. There has been no legislation that your doctor has to do amniocentesis, even if the indications are present for the procedure. (For example, I doubt you would be asked to sign a consent form saying that you were offered amniocentesis and refused, for a doctor probably cannot yet be sued for malpractice if he or she has not performed the procedure.) Your doctor should, however, *inform* you of the need, and your decision will be recorded on your chart.

Many changes are under way in this field and many top-level discussions are currently taking place as to the mandatory role of prenatal testing in obstetric care. We are probably far from reaching a point where amniocentesis would be used as a general screening program. The public is not yet widely educated about the balance between benefits of the procedure and risks involved. So it is still very much a voluntary decision, on the principle that any prenatal test will be explained to you sympathetically and honestly, leading to your own decision.

In a field such as that of congenital defects, always highly emotional, very explorative, and open to new research, where new knowledge is being gained at a rapid rate, and where the issues are often controversial, I cannot predict what the legal trends over mass genetic screening are likely to be in the near future. But it is fair to say that both amniocentesis and ultrasound have been nationally accepted as safe and good methods of detecting congenital abnormalities.

Whether a doctor is to be considered negligent if you are not informed about these tests still has to be left to the courts to decide. If you have been seeing a specialist during your pregnancy, either an obstetrician or a GP who does many deliveries, then I think you should expect such a skilled person to advise you of the availability of these tests. The decision to go ahead and have the tests and, ultimately, whether to terminate the pregnancy if a defect is found, will rest with you. Individual choice must be maintained.

*If you had X rays or took antibiotics while you were
pregnant, should you have amniocentesis?*

From time to time a woman will ask whether she ought to
have amniocentesis because of something that happened to her
in pregnancy which has made her afraid for her baby's health.
As I discussed in the previous sections, these questions are
more likely to come from mothers under thirty-five, because
they do not ordinarily fall into one of the categories indicating
the need for amniocentesis. And, while I appreciate how anxious a time pregnancy can be, particularly if you feel you have
been exposed to some chemical or environmental hazard that
could lead to your baby's being born with a defect, do let me
reassure you of the very slight risk there is of such exposure
causing harm to your fetus.

I particularly want you to appreciate this general optimistic
view, because there is no way amniocentesis can pick up damaged genes caused by environmental toxins. Even if you had
been in a nuclear explosion such as the ones in Japan in World
War II, the gene mutations that were caused by the nuclear
fallout would not show up in results from amniotic fluid culture. All that can be detected from amniocentesis is damage to
chromosomes, leading to abnormalities or biochemical problems in the fetus that might cause other specific diseases. Actual genes that have been transformed by an environmental
hazard are far too minuscule for the scientist to see, even under great magnification, and we cannot detect yet whether there
has been any genetic damage.

So, whether your particular fear relates to X rays, radiation
from nuclear plants, Love Canal–type toxins, exhaust gases,
pesticides, or caffeine, remember the individual effects cannot
be seen. If there is real cause for concern, your doctor, especially if he or she is particularly skilled in the use of ultrasound,
will check you by ultrasound in the second trimester for any

structural damage to the fetus that can be spotted on the screen. Or you may be referred to one of the special ultrasound centers, such as those at Mount Sinai in New York or Yale in New Haven. Even then, as I have indicated elsewhere, because of the insidious effect of some environmental hazards, we still cannot promise to detect every possible birth defect in the unborn fetus. So please do not feel your doctor has been negligent if, even after all the tests, your baby is unfortunately born with some damage or slight abnormality. Such incidences are very rare and you must not worry about the possibility if yours is an average, normal, healthy pregnancy.

One of the new directions of medical research, you might be interested to know, is toward solving this genetic problem. Currently work is being done to determine whether you have any harmful genes among the thousands that are attached to each chromosome. It is a development of the future, as so far we do not know what each gene controls in the body. No one can say, "This gene gives you blue or brown eyes, and this gene gives you curly or straight hair." One day, when such information is available, then maybe we will also be able to say, "This gene which directs the type of limbs in your child is now defective," and preventive measures can be taken.

Is there an alternative to amniocentesis, without penetrating the uterus?

Many thousands of women have now had amniocentesis and reports are coming back on their experiences. How does the mother feel about the benefits of the procedure compared to the risks she fears to the pregnancy? The news is not altogether good. Some women do not like the procedure. They fear that it will automatically encourage premature labor, that the needle going into the uterus will harm the fetus, and that it must hurt. These women cannot believe, however much their doctors try to reassure them, that the risks of the procedure are minimal and that to plunge a needle into the abdomen is actually going to do a pregnancy more good than harm.

Basically, no one likes to penetrate a uterus in pregnancy. And, in fact, in all branches of medicine we are turning away from invasive procedures wherever we can. But there is still no way of doing chromosomal analysis on the fetus before birth without taking an amniotic fluid sample.

I am aware that some women have negative feelings about amniocentesis, and there is new research under way at present into other methods of extracting the information without invading the mother's body. I would like to take this opportunity to bring you up to date on the latest research methods.

One new method of obtaining fetal cells without invading the uterus involves taking blood from the mother's arm (as in an ordinary blood test) and separating from it the fetal blood cells, which can then be used for chromosomal analysis. Light is reflected off the chromosomes in cells, and, incredibly, out of the million or so cells flowing through the mother's blood sample, the fetal cells can be detected by the researchers. In fact, the detection is done by computer, as the fetal chromosomes are so very different from the mother's. However, there are problems with this method. For example, the fetal cells found in the maternal blood may have come from a previous pregnancy.

Another area that has been looked at is the possibility of examining the fetal cells that may filter down from the amniotic fluid into the membranes. These could be collected in a method similar to a Pap smear.

Another noninvasive method that may become relied upon more heavily in the future will be the use of high-resolution ultrasound machines. As I have already mentioned, there are now ultrasound machines that enable us even to see movement of the baby's eyelids and pupils in the middle trimester. As work progresses to improve ultrasound, perhaps one day we

will be able to watch the whole of fetal development throughout the pregnancy—and leave nothing to guesswork.

How is amniocentesis performed?

Amniocentesis is usually done in the fourth month of pregnancy at about the sixteenth or seventeenth week (14 or 15
weeks from conception). The timing is important because at that
point of the pregnancy it is possible to extract 30 milliliters of
amniotic fluid from the relatively large total of 150 milliliters
present in the uterus at 17 weeks. The sample of amniotic fluid
can be taken without harming the fetus or the pregnancy and
it is rapidly replaced by the fetus and your body.

It might be easier and better for the mother's state of mind
to do the test earlier, but it really is not possible, since there
is not sufficient fluid to permit its safe withdrawal from the
uterus until the fourth month. And, if the test is done any later
than the seventeenth week, a problem arises over the remaining length of the pregnancy. The time between amniocentesis
being possible and when a fetus becomes legally viable, is only
about 6 to 7 weeks. Since the amniotic fluid culture takes at
least 3 weeks to grow, if it fails the first time and must be
repeated, there is scarcely time for the second results to come
in and for a termination to be done, if it should be necessary.

The appointment for amniocentesis will be made soon. There
is no difficulty in getting appointments within a few days (it is
partly to ensure this that the numbers of amniocenteses performed is restricted). You should have your husband or a good
friend along with you for the test if you are nervous, but you
do not necessarily need a companion.

In most major teaching centers, amniocentesis is performed
under ultrasound screening. This has decreased the number of
complications that can arise since it minimizes the danger that
your doctor will hit either the placenta or the baby with the

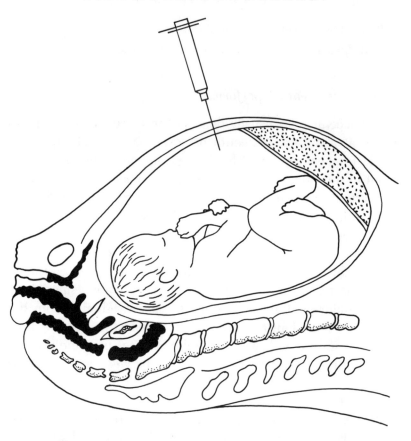

The needle in an amniocentesis procedure punctures the mother's abdominal wall, the uterus, and the amniotic sac at a point where ample fluid can easily and safely be drawn.

amniocentesis needle. The scan has to be done at the same time as the amniocentesis because, even if you had ultrasound to place the baby and placenta, say the day before, the fetus would no doubt have changed its position by the time of the amniocentesis. The ultrasound scan will also tell your doctor if the baby's size is correct for the purported stage of your pregnancy (which indicates whether your dates are right) and where the placenta is located. The doctor will also be able to see whether there is a multiple pregnancy, and if there are any visible deformities of the uterus or the fetus. Following the procedure the baby's condition is checked, which is very reassuring. So, as you can see, the use of an ultrasound scan before amniocentesis is of great benefit to both you and your doctor.

There are no special preparations necessary for amniocentesis. You can eat and drink whatever you want before coming to the hospital (and after the procedure), but you will be asked to empty your bladder before the amniocentesis is performed.

The ultrasound and amniocentesis do not have to take place in a hospital. If your doctor has his or her own ultrasound machine, it is quite in order for the procedure to be done in the doctor's own office. However, even if you do go to a hospital for the procedure, you will probably be there for less than an hour. An overnight stay is never involved. All that is entailed is for you to lie down on a table, your abdomen will be exposed, and a film of mineral oil will be rubbed over it to create a medium for the sound waves to pass through.

You will be able to watch the picture yourself on the screen. The physician will then scrub his or her hands and put on sterile gloves.

You may or may not be given a shot of local anesthetic in the skin before the amniocentesis needle is inserted. Most doctors do not give the anesthetic, as it really only means you will be stuck with a needle twice instead of once.

All you may feel is a pinch in the skin and then a cramp or pressure in the uterus as the needle passes through the uterine wall. Once it is in the fluid, the doctor withdraws the stylette from the inside of the needle and the amniotic fluid flows freely. About 30 milliliters is aspirated into a container. The needle is then slowly withdrawn. Amniotic fluid is a pale yellow color, like urine. Once the fluid has been tapped, the sonographer will switch on the ultrasound machine again and show you that your baby is alive and well.

That really is all there is to it. Except that the fluid has to get to the laboratory and most doctors ask you to take it there. That way you can be sure it will not get lost. No one wants to have to repeat the procedure because of an error like misplacing the container of fluid!

You may carry on normally afterward, but it is best not to do anything too strenuous. Why not encourage your husband to take you out to lunch? Most women find the procedure not at all worrying or painful. And that comes as a pleasant surprise.

You will have to wait at least 3 weeks to learn the results of the amniocentesis, so do not be too impatient. Why does it take so long for the results to come through? The cells in the fluid have to be grown like seeds over a period of weeks. At some point the cells are crushed, spread out and, with the use of a microscope, the chromosomes are identified and their normality is checked. The presence of the 2 sex cells also indicates the baby's sex.

Why does the culture of cells in the fluid sometimes fail, necessitating a repeat amniocentesis, and how likely is this to happen to you?

First let me say that the success rate is remarkably high.

Like the plant seeds you buy in a packet, some will grow while others refuse to take. In a similar way, the fetal cells might just not grow. Or, maybe there were not enough cells in this particular sample of fluid. Or, the mere attempt at growing cells outside of the body can produce its own aberrations. It is unfortunate when, for one of these reasons, your amniocentesis has not proved successful, for by this time you might be as much as 20 or 22 weeks pregnant, and there is a certain urgency about repeating the procedure and getting results before the pregnancy reaches 24 weeks.

However, the success rate is 98 percent with a single sample of at least 10 milliliters of fluid (30 milliliters is usually taken, to increase the number of fetal cells present). If the fluid tap is absolutely clear, then the success rate is very high—nearly 100 percent. But I know, of course, that if you are one of the 1 or 2 percent whose results are not successful, no statistics will make you feel better.

If your doctor knows you are carrying twins or, more surprisingly, discovers the multiple pregnancy on the ultrasound picture, you will be able to see the division of the two amniotic sacs on the ultrasound screen—which should be exciting for you. How is amniocentesis done on twin pregnancies? A little dye is injected into the first amniotic sac after the fluid has been tapped, and the fluid in the second sac remains free of dye. The dye is harmless and it precludes wasted repetition of the cultures.

What are the risks of amniocentesis?

You might think I have been avoiding this issue. However, as I have repeated often, amniocentesis has to be weighed for its benefits against its disadvantages. However slight the risks, amniocentesis is a surgical procedure and carries some potential dangers. So let me explain them to you.

The main danger to the mother herself is the possibility of amniocentesis introducing some infection into the amniotic fluid. This happens less than once in 1,000 women tested, but it does emphasize why it is important for the amniocentesis to be well performed by a skilled doctor, who preferably is constantly doing the procedure, because the introduction of infection is easily eliminated by good technique.

If you are an Rh-negative mother, you will be given a small dose of Rhogam after amniocentesis (see page 120).

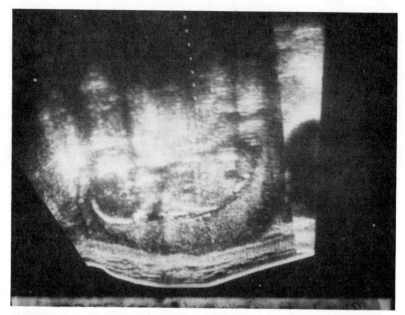

FIG. A.

FIG. B.

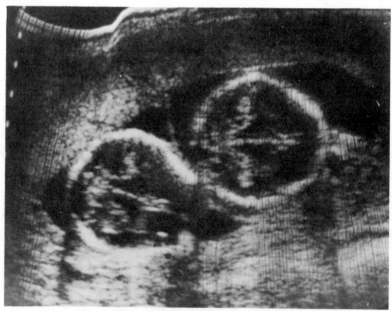

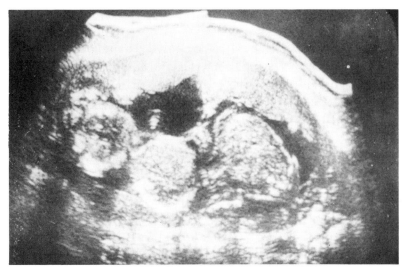

FIG. C.

FIG. A. An ultrasound picture in the second trimester shows an 18 week old fetus: the baby's head is to the left of the picture, and the small dot to the right is the baby's bladder already formed.

FIG. B. Ultrasound shows a twin pregnancy, with two fetal heads and two amniotic sacs.

FIG. C. An ultrasound picture of triplets, showing three fetal heads and three amniotic sacs.

Yale University Medical School, Dept. of Ob/Gyn, Perinatal Unit.

The one question most often asked is about the needle hitting the baby, and whether any serious damage could happen that would ruin the pregnancy or harm the baby. There have been some cases of minor scarring of tissue or skin, which may leave a small dimple on the baby's skin after birth. But, these cases are so rare and their long-term effects are in fact negligible even if the dimple stays with the child for its first few years of life, that it really is not worth worrying about. The danger of actually puncturing the fetus is eliminated by the use of ultrasound so the doctor can see where he or she is actually introducing the needle.

There is one problem that may arise after amniocentesis over which there has been some controversy. The question is whether the miscarriage rate is increased by amniocentesis and, if so, whether this means that the procedure does encourage contractions to start or the membranes to rupture. (There is, by the way, a new drug called ritodrine [see page 215], which can be safely given in very-high-risk pregnancies to stop labor where there is a real threat of its premature onset.) Controlled studies have compared the second-trimester miscarriage rate of those who have had amniocentesis and those who have not. And no difference has been found. In fact, we now say that the risk of miscarriage after amniocentesis is 0.5 percent, which is the same risk that there is for a middle-trimester miscarriage anyway.

If you do decide to terminate the pregnancy now, how difficult and painful will it be?

Obviously no one really wants to dwell beforehand on the prospect of having to terminate a pregnancy at this stage. And, of course, the vast majority of amniocentesis results are good news—providing the parents with untold relief, rather than anxiety. But if a fear of prospective termination is giving you problems before the results come through, I would like to re-assure you that the procedure involved will not be awful or painful.

Most parents who arrive for an amniocentesis will already have discussed their feelings and reached their decision about what they will do if their baby is discovered to be suffering from some incurable disease such as Down's syndrome, anencephaly, or Tay-Sachs—which will mean the baby will die shortly after birth, or, if it lives, that life will be extremely difficult for you, for the child, and for any siblings.

I do know, as must any doctor who is also a parent, how painful such decisions are. By the time you get the results from the amniocentesis you will be in the fifth, or beginning of the sixth, month of your pregnancy. The baby may be kicking and you two will have begun to establish a relationship. Because of this relationship, some women express their fears and wonder whether they would feel better by letting the pregnancy go to term, delivering normally, and then accepting that the child will not live for perhaps more than a few days, or be prepared to care for it.

I do not want to get involved in a political controversy, other than in my role as obstetrician. The decision to go ahead with a termination will have to be made by you and your husband once you have all the facts.

So, if a middle-trimester abortion is called for, you will get sympathetic support from your obstetrician and from all those who love and care for you. As I described in Chapter 1 (see page 19) in the section on induced abortion, a termination of pregnancy between 18 and 24 weeks is one in which you will be put into a mini-labor. You will be hospitalized for 1 or 2 days. Your contractions will be brought on by an intra-amniotic drug injection that puts you in labor 1 to 2 hours later and, after a variable amount of time, from 8 to 36 hours, you will deliver the fetus.

The fetus expelled will be much smaller than it would be at term, weighing less than 1 pound. So vaginally it will cause much less discomfort. Remember, too, this is still long before the legal limit when a fetus is said to be viable, or able to survive independent of the uterus. The other point to bear in mind is that the abortion will not affect your future childbearing, any more than would normal labor.

The pain involved for you should be negligible as you can be given any sedative to make the passage easier. In ordinary labor, your obstetrician is limited in helping you by what is safe for the baby. The fetus, I must emphasize, will not be left to die. Doctors are not unsympathetic, cruel people, but concerned human beings who are aware of the lifelong problems the birth of a defective or deformed child can bring to your family. If your pregnancy is terminated now, the fetus will not be alive at the moment of delivery.

If you turn back to Chapters 1 and 2, you can read there in greater depth what I have said about dealing with the psychological and emotional pressures to be suffered because of such a loss. You will have to work through feelings of sadness, of failure, of guilt at having produced a defective baby. But once you have returned to your old optimistic self, with the help of a genetics counselor and a sympathetic and understanding obstetrician, you and your husband will be able to go on to another pregnancy secure in the knowledge that most likely your next baby will be healthy and normal.

No one will ever force you to terminate a middle-trimester pregnancy, even if it is discovered that your baby has some serious abnormality. If, for any reason, you are afraid of coercion, remember that the positive side of amniocentesis is not that it encourages people to terminate pregnancies but rather the opposite. The practice of amniocentesis is persuading many couples that they can have healthy babies when, in the past, after they had given birth to one baby with a congenital abnormality, they would have been too frightened ever to conceive again in case it should happen a second time. Couples who have suffered once can now feel secure that they will not have to again. They need give birth only to healthy babies in the future.

Is there a specific screening test for spina bifida?

Many women tell me about their fears of the birth defect called spina bifida. Sometimes a woman will have a friend who has given birth to a spina bifida baby, or perhaps she lives in an area where a large proportion of such babies are born. What can she do? Is there a routine screening test to tell whether a fetus is free of this condition?

If you are going to have amniocentesis in a major genetics center for any of the reasons described in the previous sections, the fluid will automatically be tested for evidence of spina bifida or any of the neural tube defects.

But if you are not in this category, then you must know that in America today we do *not* have a routine screening test. In Britain there is a routine blood test for spina bifida. But there are several good reasons why it makes more sense there than it does here.

First let me explain about neural tube defects and the relevant test. If you remember what I said in Chapter 1 about why you must be so careful even before you know you are pregnant as to what drugs you take into your body, you will be aware that the most dangerous time for fetal development is in the first 4 weeks of life from conception (6 weeks of pregnancy), by which time the fetus's brain, spinal cord, and nervous system have all been formed. Any environmental or genetic factor that could have damaged the fetal brain and nervous system development will have come into play early in pregnancy (see page 10).

We can assess for any of these defects by measuring the amount of a protein, called alpha-fetoprotein (AFP), in the amniotic fluid or in the mother's blood (see page 166).

AFP is normally present in all pregnant women. We know that it is at its highest level at the eighteenth week of pregnancy. So if we take a blood test from the mother's arm at that time, we can determine whether the AFP level is abnormally high. Such is the routine screening test for neural tube defects.

If it is so inexpensive and simple (hardly anything is easier than a blood test, after all), why do we not do it on all pregnant women to relieve them of this fear? Well, there is a problem involved, of course. This time it is with assessing what a raised AFP level really means. The most serious cause of the rise of this chemical in the mother's blood would indeed be a neural tube defect in her baby. But there are other reasons why an

AFP reading can be very high: The dates you gave the doctor for the beginning of the pregnancy may not in fact have been correct and, if the baby is really further developed than you both imagined, the AFP level will appear high; or, you may have a multiple pregnancy that had not been spotted so far; or, you may have viral hepatitis; or a miscarriage may be imminent. All of these are more common than neural tube defects. Any of these reasons could give an abnormally high reading of AFP in your blood, leading to fear and panic until amniocentesis can be performed and then 3 or more weeks of agony waiting for the results. The only true test of AFP levels is by amniocentesis. These very seldom give what we call a "false positive."

As you can perhaps imagine, routine blood test screening of AFP would result in many more women undergoing amniocentesis for fear their baby had a neural tube defect. The figures at present stand that about 40 women out of 1,000 would have an elevated AFP reading from a blood test, which is a high percentage. But the actual figure for incidence of neural tube defects is only 1 in 1,000. So, upwards of 40 women would have to undergo amniocentesis, terrified that something was wrong with their babies, when in fact maybe 12 were really carrying twins and the others had raised AFP levels for other reasons.

Why then is the test routinely done in Britain? For some reason that we still do not understand, the incidence of neural tube defects is considerably higher in Britain than it is here. The rate there is 4.5 babies with such defects per 1,000 pregnancies; while here it is 1 per 1,000 pregnancies, which is a considerable difference. In America, neural tube defects are not as big a problem and it is felt that the cost and time taken up by screening would not be beneficial. Also, with greater use of ultrasound in the middle trimester, many defects can be picked up visually. If, however, you are at all concerned and you are not going to have amniocentesis, do request an ultrasound scan to be reassured that your baby is all right. Anyone who has had a previous child with a neural tube defect should have her blood checked as a precautionary measure, since there is unfortunately a 5 percent recurrence rate in future pregnancies.

How do we test for sickle-cell anemia and beta-thalassemia?

In discussing amniocentesis and what it *cannot* tell us, I mentioned disorders such as sickle-cell anemia and beta-thalessemia (Cooley's anemia), which are undetectable in the amniotic fluid culture. The reason we cannot find out if your baby is suffering from such diseases, from the cells grown after amniocentesis, is that researchers need a sample of the baby's blood to make these tests. How is a doctor going to get a sample of your baby's blood while it is in your uterus, you might well ask?

I would like to describe to you a very new technique that you are not likely to come across in a normal pregnancy, called *fetoscopy*. It is still a research technique available only at major teaching centers such as Yale. But, using fetoscopy, the trained obstetrician can take a sample of blood from one of the tiny vessels on the placental surface, or a sample of tissue from the baby's scalp—while the fetus remains in your uterus and without harming the pregnancy. It is difficult and still very much a research procedure.

Fetoscopy is both preceded and followed by an ultrasound scan to determine the position of the baby, the placenta, and the uterine wall. After the initial scan, the mother is given a local anesthetic on the side of the abdomen that has been selected. The obstetrician then inserts into the uterus an endoscope (a metal tube the size of a large needle used to draw blood from your arm), which has a fiber-optic light source at one end. The transparent amniotic fluid is thus illuminated, enabling inspection of the placenta and fetus. A tiny needle is then directed through the endoscope, and a sample of fetal blood from a blood vessel or a small piece of fetal skin is extracted. This method is, so far, the nearest we have come to being able to see and touch the fetus *in utero*. And as I noted before, one of the biggest frustrations for the obstetrician has always been the concealed, invisible, and unreachable presence of the baby during all those important months of its life.

You will have some idea of the difficulty of this technique if you try to imagine that the obstetrician working with the endoscope is in a position very similar to someone pressed up flat against the wall of a barn trying to see the whole wall or barn from that angle. Not only that, but it is very difficult to judge the required position of the needle in order to pierce one of the placenta's tiny veins to take a sample of blood. This is not an undertaking for every doctor and may, in fact, never develop beyond use for very selected cases in specialized units.

Fetoscopy is not, however, painful. The needle is quickly withdrawn and the mother is left to rest awhile. It can be done from the eighteenth week of pregnancy and, if a fetal tissue sample, called a biopsy, is taken, the chromosomal condition can be determined within 3 to 7 days! So if, for example, a test for Down's syndrome is required and time is imperative, fetoscopy may give results within a week rather than in the slightly more than 3 weeks called for with amniocentesis. The presence of hemophilia can also be tested by fetoscopy.

Both sickle-cell anemia and Cooley's anemia are detectable from a fetal blood sample taken in fetoscopy. Unfortunately, there is no known treatment or cure for either condition and the parents must choose whether to terminate the pregnancy if the results are positive. This can, however, be of great value to those parents who have previously had a child born with a severe defect. As both these disorders are genetically inherited, each pregnancy carries a 1 in 4 chance of producing a baby that has the disease.

There are some risks associated with fetoscopy. These have

not yet been extensively scientifically reported, as so few procedures have been done. There appears to be an increase in the abortion rate and of premature labor after fetoscopy. But, obviously, the women who will be given fetoscopy should appreciate and fully understand the cost/benefit ratio before they undergo the procedure.

Will every pregnant woman have an ultrasound scan?

Ultrasound has made major improvements in modern obstetrics. It has become incredibly valuable to doctors, as we now have a way of looking inside the uterus to see just what is developing. Much of the guesswork has gone and scientific method is aiding our clinical judgment.

Despite the obvious advantages of ultrasound, it is still not done routinely in pregnancy. Nor has it been legislated that ultrasound should be a mandatory part of prenatal care. There are problems with its cost as a screening measure for every pregnancy. Some doctors are not comfortable with its use, nor are they all trained. And as I have said before, skill and experience are vital in interpreting the pictures. Misinterpretation can lead to major errors of judgment. However, training for doctors and technicians is now offered at major teaching centers, and more and more persons are becoming accustomed to its use. I believe ultrasound scans will soon play an even more important role in prenatal care and during labor.

For now, what are the indications for doing an ultrasound scan? There are many, and I will deal with the more obvious. First, to locate the fetus and placenta prior to amniocentesis. Ultrasound is used to stage a pregnancy, as dates of a last period can be notoriously unreliable. You may have conceived during the absence of periods, or you may have been taking infertility treatment and have no idea of the date of your last period; in either case your doctor will have no real way of knowing how mature the baby is. If your labor should have to be induced because of a medical disorder such as hypertension, or if you are to have an elective caesarean and the doctor is unsure of the baby's age, then ultrasound can help in determining when the fetus will be mature enough for a safe delivery.

What can ultrasound show in the second trimester?

If you have too much or too little amniotic fluid, your doctor will want to investigate various possible causes. The presence of too much amniotic fluid need not mean anything crucial in terms of life or death. It can be a sign of a multiple pregnancy, of a blockage in the baby's gastrointestinal tract, or of a defect in the baby's nervous system.

If you have any bleeding in the second trimester, ultrasound helps your doctor rule out a condition known as *placenta previa*, in which the placenta is implanted in the lower part of the uterus. Placenta previa at term means you must be delivered by caesarean section. But there is no need for panic if placenta previa is discovered in the second trimester, as a large percentage of such low placentas somehow migrate to a normal position later in pregnancy. And at least a cause will have been found for the bleeding.

If placenta previa is found, then another ultrasound will be done later in the pregnancy to confirm the position. Research work at Yale has very recently devised a method of grading the placenta according to its appearance at different stages of pregnancy. This can also be used as a help in assessing the baby's maturity.

Even the baby's sex may be predicted from an ultrasound picture, though this is seldom a reason for having ultrasound. The method is no more sophisticated than seeing if the fetus has a penis or not! It is not always an accurate method, and you might be in for a surprise or a shock at birth—so do not paint the nursery based on that information. (The amniocentesis sex confirmation is, however, accurate.)

Finally, if you are ever wondering just how your baby is doing even though you feel its kicks and movements, then an ultrasound scan will be able to give you and your doctor lots of information on its general well-being. We call this a *biophysical* program; it is a system of checking for various signs that indicate a healthy baby. For example, your doctor will check to see how the baby moves in reaction to the ultrasound waves, or to pressure on your abdomen. He or she will also watch the baby's breathing movements, check on whether the volume of amniotic fluid is evenly distributed through the amniotic cavity, and see how the baby uses its limbs and the way it holds its head. Such a test is quick and very accurate. It really is a good idea for your doctor to begin monitoring fetal well-being in the second trimester (particularly if you have some medical disorder such as high blood pressure), even though such work is generally reserved for the third trimester. (See pages 226–239 for much more on the assessment of fetal well-being.)

How safe is ultrasound?

Ultrasound is made up of high-frequency sound waves that cannot be heard by the human ear. The sound waves are produced by electrical energy. They are emitted from a transducer in the ultrasound machine and, as they pass through human tissue, they rebound at each surface and return to the machine, where they create an image. Since it contains no ionizing radiation, ultrasound is nothing like an X ray, which might induce structural damage in the baby. It is really very beneficial to the management of the pregnancy and will not harm the baby or you. Repeat ultrasounds are safe and quite normal. Over a million women each year have at least one scan in pregnancy, and this number will no doubt increase as many doctors are now doing routine scans. According to the latest reports, there has been no sign of harm to patients or to babies from ultrasound. Research is continuing to establish safety limits.

Sometimes I am asked if there is any danger in the machine's being left running while the doctor is talking to you. The answer is that the machine is not left running, though you may think it is. When the doctor is taking time to explain the pictures to you, although the machine is on, the emission of sound waves has been turned off, and the picture has been frozen. Ultrasound must of course be used intelligently, but I hope you will be reassured by the positive results of research into its safety. The very fact that you are not required to sign a consent form before ultrasound shows that there is no official recognition of any potential risk.

However, some people are anxious about the effect of ultrasound on the fetus, particularly in respect to the baby's developing auditory system; the sound waves, though, are not in the audible range. If you so wish, you may decline to have the ultrasound tests. If you make such a decision, you should be aware that in fact the Fetone, with which your doctor and you can hear the baby's heartbeat, is potentially more dangerous than ultrasound, as it is a continuous sound beam (not pulsed). If you are going to reject ultrasound, you should also reject the use of the Fetone and request that your doctor use an ordinary stethoscope.

YOUR SECOND-TRIMESTER LIFE STYLE

Enjoy your renewed energy level in the second trimester, for by the third you will probably be feeling a lot more tired and heavy with your ever-growing abdomen. But do bear in mind the restrictions on what you eat and drink (see page 122). Caffeine should be limited to three caffeine-containing drinks a day; no soft or hard drugs or over-the-counter medications should be taken; and if possible no cigarettes and little alcohol should be consumed. The period of greatest danger, of organogenesis, is over and all your baby's organs will have been formed, but the baby now needs all the oxygen and nutrition it can get for its growth and weight gain.

Because your abdomen is getting larger, you will be wearing loosely fitting garments or maternity clothes. It is wise to think ahead to the season you will be going into, for by the third trimester you will be *much* bigger again. Do not waste money on summer clothes if the third trimester is going to be in winter. You can probably make do for now with some baggy trousers or loose dresses.

Travel

This is the best time of pregnancy in which to travel. But you will begin to notice some discomfort if you have to sit in cramped conditions for any length of time. Flying is safe and if you are going on a long flight, why not see if you can arrange ahead of time to block the seat next to you. Do not be scared to inform the airline that you are in the second trimester of pregnancy and would like a spare seat left available if it is at all possible. Sitting upright for long periods will not harm your baby, but it may become uncomfortable for you, causing back pain and stiffening sensations around the uterus. You will need to get up every hour or so and walk around the plane, to keep your circulation going and your posture from sinking into a permanent bend! For such a journey, wear very comfortable shoes that you can easily slip on and off, as your feet are likely to swell.

The same is true for a long ride by car. You will need to make regular stops, walk around, and keep your circulation going. It is advisable to make sure you have another driver with you. Do not undertake anything longer than a 3-hour drive alone in the middle trimester of pregnancy, or later. You will become more tired than usual; the isolation and concentration could make you feel anxious and panicky, neither of which reaction is good for driving.

Work

There is no reason to leave work in the second trimester, unless your doctor advises it because you are having some medical problem with the pregnancy, such as bleeding or cramping, high blood pressure, or undue swelling of the feet, hands or body; or if your weight gain is too slow, leading to suspicions of IUGR (intrauterine growth retardation); or if you are feeling so tired that extra rest is recommended. If you do continue with work, remember that you must arrange to have more rest than usual and continue with a sensible nutritious diet. It may be advisable to skip any lunch dates or parties, and to stay in your office, eating a freshly prepared salad or a whole-wheat-bread sandwich brought from home; put your feet up, for that hour or so, in order to build up strength and stamina for the afternoon. Do not expect to be able to shop and buy your maternity outfits, dashing around the stores during your lunch break. Do not try to push yourself to the limit. That will only lead to strain and the possibility of some medical problem caused by undue stress. If your job entails long hours on your feet, you should ask for a chair to sit on for most of the day. It is not wise to stand for great lengths of time in midpregnancy (or later), as it will hinder your body's circulation and you may encourage varicose veins. You will only appreciate this advice in retrospect, after you have tried resting. Give yourself some time to be selfish.

Exercise

Gentle exercises should be all right in a normal healthy pregnancy, as long as you do not suffer any bleeding or cramping.

If you begin to feel by the end of the sixth month that your body is getting too cumbersome for exercise, if you are afraid the jolting will induce premature labor or that your breathlessness might be doing the baby some harm, do not feel guilty about giving up the particular form of exercise till after the birth. You can still make sure to walk a lot in the normal course of the day.

By the beginning of the third trimester, you will probably notice a shift in your temperament again, bringing with it a desire to be calm, restful, withdrawn, and somewhat of a homebody. This appears to be caused by more than the psychological expectation of the imminent birth and hinges on changes in brain metabolism throughout pregnancy.

As you grow larger, the ideal sport is swimming, since your weight is supported by the water and you are still getting excellent cardiovascular exercise. Running, jogging, or calisthenics are permitted, but you should discuss these with your doctor first. Never take the level of exercise as high as you would in the nonpregnant state; do not push yourself to run those last few miles in extra fast time. Your body should force you to run more slowly and, by the end of the trimester, certain calisthenics exercises should be discontinued, such as those that involve lying flat on your belly. Avoid jumps or too strenuous exercises that squeeze the abdomen into strange positions. I advise you to read one of the excellent books available on the exercises that are good for you in pregnancy and are permissible right through to labor.

Many people need educating on pregnancy today and how much is possible in your life that used to be forbidden. Whether the cardiovascular exercises, such as running, aerobics, or swimming, are in any way bad for pregnancy has not yet been fully researched or scientifically documented. There have been some controversial arguments put forward that too much exertion will prevent oxygen getting through to the baby. But so far no such exercise has been associated with birth defects or with difficulties in labor. Rather the opposite: fit and athletic women often have easier labor and healthy pregnancies. You can contact the Women's Sports Foundation, 195 Moulton, San Francisco, CA 94123, for more information and current material on the subject. The WSF is a nonprofit agency aimed at educating and helping women in their pursuit of fitness.

I have described Braxton Hicks contractions (see page 158), the natural contractions the uterus makes throughout life that are only noticeable in pregnancy. They will become more obvious throughout your second trimester as your belly gets larger. Sometimes, after a period of exercising, you might notice stronger and harder contractions. As long as the contractions do not go on for too long, and are not associated with pain or the passage of blood, you can be confident that all is quite normal. They might mean you have overexerted yourself, in which case you should cut down the level of exercise. If the contractions are associated with bleeding, see your doctor immediately. If they are associated with pressure on the cervix (a mild pain in the vaginal area), stop the vigorous form of exercise immediately and inform your doctor at your next visit.

Many women begin a specific prenatal exercise class, such as those of the Lamaze school, at this time or around 28 to 30 weeks. The exercises concentrate on the lower back, lower half of the uterus, and the pelvis and perineal area (your vagina and its muscles), as well as on breathing techniques that will be a vital support in labor. Even though you feel fit and energetic, you must not overlook the benefit of such exercises and training for labor itself—and the meeting with other women at a similar stage of pregnancy can do wonders for your state of mind. Some couples prefer private classes, but it really may be better to be with other couples.

Sex

Sex should come back into your lives in the middle trimester, as your libido will once again be released, lifting the depressing qualities of the first trimester. Many pregnant women in the second trimester feel a greater sexuality than they do in normal times. The hormonal changes now create an aura of well-being. There is a glow to your cheeks. Your hair shines and looks healthy. Some women say they feel more feminine than they ever have before. You might feel fulfilled, and even blatantly sexual, with those large breasts and the budding belly that announces to the world that you are a sexual being.

Men differ in their responses to pregnant women. In the street, you may not be subjected to catcalls and wolf whistles; but, once pregnant, you do become public property, and men, as well as women, are likely to stop to talk. They want to know how pregnant you are, what you are going to call the baby. They feel happy for you and your pregnancy, as, in an oblique way, it confirms their own optimism about life.

You should have lost most of your earlier fears of sexual intercourse, although you may still worry that full intercourse will harm the baby or set off premature labor. As I explained in Chapter 2, there is very little danger in a normal healthy pregnancy of intercourse or orgasm causing a miscarriage or premature labor, and indeed many women who have suffered first-trimester miscarriages in previous pregnancies will be freed in the second trimester to enjoy sex again. However, if you have ever had a second-trimester miscarriage, you should be careful to avoid intercourse in this period. If you are at all concerned, ask your doctor when intercourse will be safe for you.

Although intercourse will not harm the baby, you will of course have to judge what position is comfortable for you. You will probably not want your husband's weight pressing down on your belly, since it might well cause undue pressure on you.

Together, you and your husband can explore different positions. Maybe now is the time to be more adventurous in sex and to bring about some long-term changes in your life. Your husband should not be shocked if you suggest trying out different positions, as he must appreciate, too, that sex in the classic man-on-top position is no longer going to be as comfortable.

If you lie on your side so your belly is supported by the bed or floor, then your husband can also lie on his side and approach you face to face. Or you can lie on your side and he can approach you from behind and enter your vagina from that position. This is often found to be one of the most comfortable and comforting positions in pregnancy, as your husband can wrap his arms around you and stroke your belly at the same time intercourse takes place. You can sit on the edge of a low bed with your husband kneeling in front of you; which will let you wrap your legs around him, leaning back on your arms. You can lie on your back, leaning on your elbows, or he can prop you with pillows, then kneel in front of you so his weight is on his arms rather than on your belly. Obviously, you can sit astride him, which, with your newly enlarged breasts, might appeal to both of you as an extra excitement.

None of these positions will be easy for you if you are ashamed of the sight of your body as it grows bigger. I know that it can be difficult to accept these changes. They are all happening so fast and you do not even recognize this mound of flesh as yourself when you stand before a mirror—so what must your husband be thinking? It is probably quite difficult *not* to have an underlying sense of shame at being so large. You have spent years coming to terms with your normal body, trying to be slim, and now you are suddenly supposed to feel comfortable with this new and, occasionally even to you, grotesque sight. However, you must both learn to love the sight of you with the belly if you are to make your sex life enjoyable during pregnancy. And, as I indicated before, where it is medically approved I do believe that an active sex life in pregnancy helps bond you and your husband to the infant before its birth. Now is the time to indulge in the *romance* of having a baby. Don't lose the opportunity.

C H A P T E R

4

The Third Trimester

28 – 40 W E E K S

The third trimester affects each woman differently. Some women feel tired, exhausted, and anxious for the birth to be over. Others continue to feel vigorous and elated as they did in the second trimester. They remain active and optimistic and prefer not to think about that anxiety-making time known as labor. Whatever your frame of mind, there is really no need for any fear. Your doctor will be checking you regularly now: every 2 weeks until the thirty-sixth week and then once a week until the birth. Most of your doctor's attention in this trimester will be concerned with monitoring the baby's growth to ensure it is receiving an adequate supply of oxygen and food (glucose) from the placenta.

Today many tests are available to judge the baby's health—which we term "fetal well-being"—and your doctor will discuss with you at each stage just what is being done and why. None of the tests includes intervention in the uterus, as did the major tests of the second trimester, so you can rest assured that there is little danger involved for either you or the baby.

The fetus is viable from 28 weeks and could be born with a

good chance of survival. If by chance the environment in your uterus is no longer beneficial for the baby, then your doctor may choose to induce an early birth, rather than risk any problem that might occur in a prolonged pregnancy; this is where the phrase "better out than in" becomes applicable. The obstetrician's main concern is to ensure that letting your baby go to term is the best possible course both for the child and for you. But you will be reading a lot more about how the doctor makes such a judgment as this chapter continues. In the average normal pregnancy no judgments have to be made. Watchful expectancy is the order of the day.

What changes are happening to the mother?

If your response to the third trimester is to feel very anxious and to wish you could have the baby now and get it over with, do not feel concerned that this indicates a less than motherly attitude, or that it might indicate something is wrong with the baby. The anxiety, or sense of urgency, you are experiencing is not only psychological; it also probably occurs because a metabolic change takes place in the brain in this trimester.

Subtle shifts have gone on in each trimester, bringing about the depression and fatigue of the first, the elation and vigor of the second, and now the anxiety of the third. Most women experience these trimester shifts in their emotional outlook. We have just not known why until very recently. Brain metabolism is a new area of research and there will soon be more information on this development.

If this is your first pregnancy you will probably be more anxious about the birth than will a woman who has had previous children. Birth itself is a leap into the dark for the first-time mother. How will you know when you are in labor? Will you get to the hospital on time? Will labor be painful? Will you be able to do the breathing when it comes to it? These are all nagging questions that can obsess the mind in the third trimester.

You will probably begin to feel very dependent on your husband, on a close friend or family member. I encourage you to talk about your fears as much as you need to to such a person, and to your doctor. Remember, your obstetrician knows how you are feeling right now. He or she should be prepared to spend time listening to you and reassuring you.

The baby is growing rapidly now, at the rate of about a pound a week, and you will begin to put on weight in a way you have so far not experienced. Your belly will protrude so much that some people will assume you are about to give birth in the supermarket or the theater, and not in 2 months time. As your abdomen grows you may experience some swelling of the feet, particularly in hot weather. If you lie on your back for too long you may feel some faintness, known as supine-hypotension, which can be relieved by rolling over onto your side.

Sleep may become a problem if you get too big, as no position in bed is comfortable. Lying on your side is best, with one knee up to the chest and the other knee stretched out, your arms over your head. This will take some pressure off the abdomen. If your baby kicks a lot during the night, it can cause insomnia for you, which may make you irritable from lack of sleep. Try to view this discomfort positively; it's the surest test of fetal well-being there is. Sedatives are not recommended even for chronic insomnia, as they make the baby sleepy too.

Do not underestimate the tension of waiting and worrying on your emotional relationships, particularly with your husband. It is not a good time to be having serious quarrels at home, though it is unfortunately quite common for them to occur. Both of you will be feeling the responsibility of the birth weighing upon you and the fear of changes in your life style— which may be expressed in irritability. (Most of these tensions will be released by the drama of the birth itself, and you and your husband will be drawn together.) A very serious quarrel may help to set off labor early, though it is doubtful that it will bring on premature labor unless other, physical conditions are preparing the baby for exit at this time. (If you go into labor any time after 37 weeks, it is not considered premature.)

If you begin to feel more and more short of breath as pregnancy advances, this should slacken off during the last month, making life more comfortable for you from the thirty-sixth week as the baby descends into the pelvis at this stage. However, as you will read below, descent and engagement do not necessarily occur till after labor commences, so you cannot *rely* on their happening.

It is not uncommon for you to develop low backache or pain in the lower abdomen (in the pubic region) during the third trimester. This is due to an alteration in the center of gravity of the body because of the enlarged uterus, plus the slight loosening of the pelvic joints, probably owing to the hormone relaxin, which softens pelvic ligaments to allow expansion for childbirth. To help prevent backache, sit with a straight back, do not slouch, and do not wear high-heeled shoes. Sit in a hard chair or on the floor. Always bend with a straight back or, if lifting, bend from the knees and lift from a crouching position.

Colostrum usually begins to appear from the nipples during the third trimester. Its early excretion is a good sign and is due to the changing hormonal levels in preparation for the birth. You should now begin to wash the nipples carefully, and oil them with something gentle like baby lotion if they are becoming hard and cracked. You can also gently massage and exercise the nipples, pulling them forward to encourage the later secretion of milk into the breast.

You will probably pass urine more often as the enlarged uterus presses on the bladder. You may be constipated at this time, so eat lots of fresh fruit and vegetables, and drink plenty of fluids. You will probably not feel as hungry during the last few weeks of pregnancy and there is no need to eat heavily, as the baby will get sufficient nourishment from the placenta.

Concentrate on a diet of fresh foods, salads, protein, and as little carbohydrate as necessary. Your weight may even begin to fall in the last month of pregnancy or just stabilize, as the amount of amniotic fluid manufactured is much less. The baby is now so big, it takes up most of the space in the amniotic sac and less fluid is produced.

You will perspire a lot and get very hot—which is fine in winter as it keeps you warm, but can make summer living, especially in big steamy cities, quite uncomfortable. The reason for the perspiration and heat is that you are in a hypermetabolic state, which basically means your body is working at full steam and you are producing everything at maximum.

Of course I should advise you to get your overnight bag packed well before the visit to the hospital, but somehow I do not feel you need reminding of that obvious fact. If you have other children, be prepared with emergency measures for taking care of them, as babies have a habit of arriving when least expected and often in the middle of the night. If you end up rushing to the hospital having grabbed only your coat and without even time to pick up your toothbrush, never mind. It is not going to spoil your experience of labor and delivery, and your husband or a relative can always bring your cosmetics and nightgown to you later. Once labor is over and you have your baby in your arms, such matters seem very inconsequential.

What changes are happening to the baby?

Twenty-sixth week after conception (which compares to the twenty-eighth week of traditional pregnancy dating): The fetus is viable and can live separately, independently, and, if born, has to be registered. There is a legal controversy now about the term *viability*, as these days, with good neonatal care, a fetus has a chance of surviving even at 26 weeks. Traditional limits were set years ago when medicine was not as advanced as it is now. At 28 weeks, the survival rate can be as high as 70 percent, depending on the hospital where you deliver (unfortunately, intensive neonatal care units are only found in major teaching centers).

There are more babies being born at this early stage, probably because the drugs now used to stop premature labor can often forestall birth until around the twenty-sixth week. If a woman experiences premature labor, say as early as the twentieth week, and is put on ritodrine, that may stop the labor until this point.

At this stage, the fetus is still covered with greasy vernix, and its lungs are not mature. Its length is about 37 centimeters (14¾ inches) and its weight is around 900 grams (2 pounds).

Thirtieth week after conception: The baby is now perfectly formed. The head is in proportion to the body and the baby has a good chance of survival if born. The baby is about 40.5 centimeters (16 inches) long and weighs about 1.6 kilograms (3½ pounds).

Thirty-sixth week after conception: The baby is now considered fully mature, meaning its organs are not only formed but working normally. It can survive if born, or if it has to be delivered by induction or caesarean section, there is a lesser problem with lung maturity, since the lungs are now prepared for respiration outside the mother's body. The baby will be about 46 centimeters (18 inches) long, and will weigh around 2½ kilograms (5½ pounds).

Thirty-eighth week after conception: The baby is ready to be born. The fine body hair called *lanugo* has disappeared, and the baby has early head hair. Its eyes will be blue (all babies are born with blue eyes, though the color may well change a few weeks after birth). The nails are properly grown. It will have put on a lot of fat in the past month and look chubby at birth.

At term a baby might be as long as 50 centimeters (nearly 20 inches), and weigh on average 3.5 kilograms (7½ pounds). Though, of course, babies differ in weight and length.

YOUR HEALTH AND CONDITION

What your doctor is looking for in the last 2 months of pregnancy

Between 32 and 36 weeks, visits will usually be every 2 weeks; from 36 to 40 weeks, you will pay your doctor weekly visits. Your obstetrician will perform the checks for blood pressure and urine as has been done all along. Now more emphasis will be placed on the baby's position. From 36 weeks it is important to ensure that the baby's head is presenting over the pelvis (head down). Do not worry if the baby's bottom (breech) presents at 30 or 32 weeks, as this occurs in 25 percent of women and the baby turns on its own as full term approaches. If the baby is still in a breech position, or in any position other than head down, by 36 or 38 weeks, and definitely by 40 weeks, your doctor will have to try to determine why. If no cause— such as a small pelvis, a fibroid, or placenta in the way—is found, he or she may try to correct the position by turning the baby (see section on external version, page 212), or decide whether you are to have a caesarean section instead of a vaginal delivery.

During the last month of pregnancy, internal examinations are done at each visit to check the cervix. Near term the cervix first shortens in length (effacement) and then may begin to dilate. If your doctor tells you you are already 1 centimeter dilated, for example, the statement will be accompanied by the news that labor might begin sometime soon. Your doctor does *not* require these frequent visits in the expectation that anything might go wrong, but so that he or she can ensure that all remains well right to the end.

The internal examination in the third trimester will not induce labor. After the exam, you may have some brown staining, which will be a small amount of blood and mucus from the plug in the cervix. In itself this is not enough to dislodge the plug, or bring on the "show" (which is a sign of the onset of labor). If you genuinely experience the show, the amount of blood and mucus will be enough to fill the palm of your hand. So do not worry about a slight stain after an examination.

If necessary, there are tests that can tell your doctor how healthy and strong the baby is during these last few weeks of pregnancy. These tests are ultrasound, fetal heart rate monitoring (stress and nonstress testing), and hormonal measurements (e.g., for estriol) in your blood (see pages 226–239).

What does vaginal bleeding in the third trimester mean?

Any loss of blood in the third trimester is known as an antepartum hemorrhage, and must be reported immediately to your doctor. It may be nothing serious, but the exact cause of the bleeding must be diagnosed. Bleeding can arise from anywhere in the genital tract. It is not uncommon for bleeding to follow intercourse at this stage of pregnancy as the cervix becomes very engorged with blood, which can lead to surface bleeding. Your doctor will examine your cervix with a speculum to see if this is the case.

An important cause of bleeding at this stage may be placenta previa (see page 192). During even normal Braxton Hicks contractions, such a placenta will become disturbed, as the lower half of the uterus is pulled up by the contraction, and this causes the bleeding. Symptoms of placenta previa usually begin around the thirtieth week, and you will have repeated little hemorrhages of bright red blood, known as "warning hemorrhages." (The blood is bright red, since it comes from so low in the uterus, near the cervix.)

In such a case, vaginal examination by hand is dangerous, since it can lead to heavy bleeding. So the confirming examination will be done by ultrasound.

If placenta previa is diagnosed at this point, the baby will be delivered by caesarean section, once it is mature. Until maturity has been established, you will be observed in the hospital in case there is any further bleeding. The blood, by the way, comes entirely from the mother and not from the baby.

Another cause of bleeding in the third trimester is known as *abruptio placentae*. This usually happens slightly later than a placenta previa, after the thirty-fifth or thirty-sixth week. The bleeding occurs from a *normally* situated placenta (in the upper part of the uterus) which separates from the uterine wall. It can be a far more serious condition for the baby, as it can mean the baby is cut off from its blood supply. It may also cause blood-clotting deficiencies in the mother, putting her at risk. Abruptio is far more difficult to diagnose than placenta previa. Usually there is no warning, but the mother may have severe abdominal pain and *dark* vaginal bleeding. If your doctor examines your abdomen and finds that the uterus is tender and hard, it may be an indication of this condition.

If abruptio placentae is diagnosed (by ultrasound), you will usually be delivered by caesarean section. When the baby is mature (beyond 36 weeks), many doctors will induce labor for an attempt at vaginal delivery. There is now new work to suggest that with skilled antepartum fetal heart rate monitoring (see pages 231–232), it is possible to wait to near term and then induce or await labor, checking frequently by various tests to make sure that the baby is not suffering any stress from an impaired placenta.

There are some cases of bleeding in the third trimester that do not fit any of these causes and remain undiagnosed. With the better diagnostic support offered by ultrasound, however, this is now a smaller group. In cases where no cause for the bleeding can be found, you will be kept in the hospital until bleeding ceases, and you will be observed more frequently by your doctor. You should refrain from further sexual intercourse.

Hypertension

If you develop hypertension in late pregnancy, you will be hospitalized and investigated. Hypertension may interfere with the functioning of the placenta and prevent it from efficiently transporting food (glucose) and oxygen to the baby.

The baby's development can also be monitored by fetal heart rate monitoring (for nonstress and stress testing, see pages 235–236). If your blood pressure is very high you may be given a drug to lower it. The baby's lung maturity will also be tested by amniocentesis. As I will explain later in this chapter, the critical point in the third trimester of a problematical pregnancy comes when your doctor must assess whether your baby is in greater danger remaining in the uterus than being cared for in the nursery. If in a case of severe hypertension the baby is being starved of oxygen and food, then induced labor may be necessary even before the baby's lungs have matured (see page 223 for treatment of the immature newborn).

What does it mean if your baby is positioned abnormally?

The normal position (presentation) for a baby at the end of pregnancy is head down, but there are a variety of other possibilities. Early in the third trimester, when there is a lot of amniotic fluid relative to the baby's size, it swims around and changes position frequently. At the thirtieth week, as many as one in four babies are in the *breech* position (the bottom over the pelvis) but usually the baby's head goes down during the course of the pregnancy, because of the baby's greater size, its heavier head, and the shape of the uterus.

Your obstetrician will therefore not be too interested in checking the baby's position until at least the thirty-fourth week. If, after the thirty-fourth week, the presentation is not normal—which your doctor can tell by checking the fetal outline externally—he or she may elect to turn the baby manually. This is known as an "external cephalic version." Your doctor can only do an external version if the circumstances are suitable (and not all doctors practice it). It should not be done if you have had a previous caesarean section, if the placenta is on the anterior wall, or if you have high blood pressure. The doctor will first check the baby's heartbeat and the position of the placenta by ultrasound. Then, the version, or turning, is performed by your doctor taking one hand to the baby's head and the other to its buttocks and gently flexing and juggling the baby around. Undue force is never used. Ultrasound will show your baby's heart beating normally after the version is completed. You will be observed at rest for an hour after the procedure. It is not painful to have an external version done, though it may cause some minor discomfort. If the doctor has real difficulties doing an external version, it may be because the uterus is too tense. Beta-mimetics are now available that will relax the uterus; these drugs are also used to stop premature labor. Using these drugs is a new development, but an obstetrician can work more effectively with a relaxed uterus.

If it is impossible to change the baby's position and prevent a breech presentation, your obstetrician will have to decide whether to deliver you by caesarean section or vaginally. Two influencing factors are the size of the baby and the size of your pelvis, both of which can be assessed clinically, often with the help of ultrasound.

Are you "big enough" for the baby?

Especially in a first pregnancy, mothers nearly always ask this question. In a well-nourished society, most women have adequately sized pelves. In impoverished populations, doctors often have to perform more caesarean sections because the women's pelves are too small. When I worked in Africa, for example, many women had such poor nutrition that their pelvic bones had not formed well and a 7- or 8-pound baby just could not get through.

A pelvic assessment by internal examination is done in late pregnancy at the same time as your doctor feels for the position of the baby's head and the condition of your cervix. If your pelvis is really too small, you may be allowed to go into labor, but you will have a caesarean section if no progress takes place. Often pleasant surprises occur even in cases where vaginal delivery seems most unlikely—the joints of the pelvis may give a little to allow stretching.

Your pelvis might be large enough for a 6-pounder, but not for an 8-pounder. If the baby has engaged, which means the widest part of the baby's head has entered the brim of the pelvis, then there should be no mechanical problem. But if the baby has not engaged (and, contrary to standard textbooks, only 50 percent do engage in women having their first baby, and only 20 percent in women with previous children), your doctor will do the simple procedure of pressing down on the abdomen to see if the baby's head will tip into the pelvis. Next an internal pelvic examination will enable the doctor to feel the bony landmarks in the pelvis at different levels. It used to be common to employ the use of X rays to measure the pelvic size. But pelvimetry using X rays is done very seldom nowadays, since we are reluctant to use X rays during pregnancy.

What problems are likely to occur with twins?

Twins are more common in older mothers, so we are probably going to see more and more of them in the future. (See below, page 216, for the use of amniocentesis to detect Down's syndrome in twins carried by older mothers.) The incidence of twins is increased if you have been taking ovulation-inducing drugs such as clomiphene (Clomid) and particularly fertility drugs given by injection (Pergonal), which result in an even higher frequency of multiple pregnancies. If you are a member of a particular ethnic group there is a difference. For white people the incidence of twins is about 1 in every 90 pregnancies, but it is much higher in the black population, where, for some unknown reason, more fraternal twins occur. In the whole population, the rate of incidence for triplets is 1 in nearly 10,000 pregnancies.

When are you likely to find out you are carrying twins? If you have an ultrasound scan early in pregnancy, either routinely or because your doctor is suspicious that you seem bigger than would normally be expected from your dates, then you might be diagnosed as early as 10 weeks. One of my patients was not sure of the date of her last period. We thought she might have been 10 weeks pregnant, and to confirm this I gave her an ultrasound scan and discovered she was carrying twins. You could actually see the two amniotic sacs and two fetal hearts (see illustration page 182).

A decade ago, twins were seldom diagnosed before 20 weeks, as only then would we be alerted by the mother suddenly appearing larger than her dates suggested. So the use of ultrasound has made a vast improvement here. It is a great advantage to diagnose a multiple pregnancy early, as the parents will have more time to become accustomed to the idea and certain medical management can be initiated.

Twin (or multiple) pregnancies are quite normal variations of the pregnant condition and there is no reason to be anxious should you find you are carrying twins. However, these pregnancies are more prone to certain complications, so it is worth knowing about them—but not worth worrying about them. The main problem is the possibility of premature labor. Generally speaking, with a twin pregnancy, labor will commence 2 or 3 weeks ahead of time. But we want to prevent it from happening any earlier than that.

Prevention of premature labor calls for more frequent visits to your doctor to check the condition of your cervix. Then, if your doctor does discover any changes that might indicate the onset of premature labor, you will be advised to take extra bed rest. It is a good idea, anyway, with a twin pregnancy, to get your feet off the ground for 2 or 3 hours a day, as this takes pressure off the cervix.

Fortunately, if premature labor is suspected—either because you feel contractions, have frequent runs of fairly intense contractions, or if your doctor sees that your cervix is beginning to shorten and open—you can be given a drug to inhibit premature labor (see page 184). This drug, ritodrine, has been proved safe for use in pregnancy and very effective. The only surviving sextuplets in the world, born in South Africa, were delivered quite miraculously near term. This was made possible by the use of a uterine relaxant drug to prevent premature labor. Ordinarily babies of such a multiple pregnancy do not have a good chance of survival because of early premature labor.

How different will the management of your pregnancy be with twins? Basically, I would say you should expect more frequent visits to your doctor and more bed rest. Some of the minor discomforts of pregnancy (nausea, heartburn, varicose veins) will be increased because of the presence of two fetuses, but not to the frightening extent you may have been led to believe. Your diet should include an extra folic acid supplement, as folic acid is necessary for tissue growth.

There are some new developments in the management of twin pregnancy I would like to tell you about. Sonographic monitoring can now help your doctor exclude a possible problem known as "twin transfusion syndrome." It is a rare condition in which twin babies share the blood supply across the placenta; as time goes on, one twin may receive the majority of the blood supply at the expense of the other (at its extreme, one twin dies). The condition can now be avoided because ultrasound will show that one of the twins is lagging behind in its growth. It may then be decided to induce the birth earlier, either vaginally or by caesarean section, to ensure two healthy babies.

The use of ultrasound also now means that an older mother carrying twins needn't have the risk of a Down's syndrome baby as she can have an amniocentesis. With the aid of ultrasound before the amniocentesis, your doctor can see the two fetal sacs. Moreover, if Down's syndrome should be discovered in just one of the twins you do not necessarily have to abort both. A recent procedure performed by my friend and colleague Dr. Thomas Kerenyi at the Mount Sinai Hospital in New York demonstrates the new possibilities. In this case one twin was normal while the other had Down's syndrome; Kerenyi was able to abort the Down's twin in the uterus by a needle insertion into the fetal sac that terminated that pregnancy, and later the mother went on to deliver one normal healthy baby to the delight of both parents.

ONSET OF LABOR

How can you tell whether you are in labor?

It can be difficult to know when you are in established labor. If you are unsure, call your doctor and discuss it with him or her. Do not be afraid of making a fool of yourself. Sometimes your doctor or his nurse may be uncertain and will ask you to come into the office or visit the labor floor to be observed and checked. Labor commences in one of three ways:

1. *Onset of contractions:* As I mentioned previously, uterine contractions occur throughout pregnancy and especially in the last trimester. These are called Braxton Hicks contractions and they differ from labor in that they occur at infrequent intervals and last a short time. Labor contractions, by definition, last longer and longer and get progressively stronger. Chemical

changes have occurred in the muscle of the uterus, and these turn it into an organ very much like the human heart, which beats all the time. If you begin to have regular contractions, lie down and time them over the course of an hour. If they get stronger and more uncomfortable and occur at intervals of 8 minutes or less from the start of one contraction to the start of another, call your doctor. Once labor is well established the contractions occur every 2 to 3 minutes and the tightening lasts from 40 to 45 seconds. At this frequency you usually cannot talk through them and may need to do your breathing exercises. Ordinarily, if you cannot decide whether your contractions mean you are in labor, you are not!

There is no extreme urgency about diagnosing the onset of labor, as you normally have many hours to get to the hospital—especially in a first pregnancy.

2. *Rupture of the membranes:* Labor may be preceded by rupture of the membranes (your water breaks), by some hours or even days. But this usually means the onset of labor contractions. If the membranes do not rupture of their own accord, or your doctor does not break them for you, classically they rupture at full dilation of the cervix and then herald the second stage of labor (the birth of the baby). You should get into bed and call your doctor if your water breaks, whether you have contractions or not. Occasionally, if the baby's head is not deep in the pelvis, there is a risk that the umbilical cord may come down, which could be dangerous.

There will usually be no question that your water has broken as there will be a continuous passage of clear fluid running from the vagina. However, if it is only a trickle, it may be difficult to diagnose. Amniotic fluid is clear, but it may be slightly blood-tinged from its passage through the plug at the cervix. It has an almond smell. Sometimes, when going to the toilet, or on returning to bed from doing so, you may involuntarily pass urine. This urinary incontinence can be from the pressure of the baby's head on the nerves surrounding the bladder. If your doctor is uncertain about what is happening, he or she will push up the baby's head when you are being examined and see if there is any leakage of amniotic fluid; or the doctor may use a litmus-paper test that will indicate whether the fluid in the vagina is acid or alkaline, as urine is acid and will not effect a color change in the paper.

If your membranes rupture near term, labor will usually ensue within a few hours. In some cases, however, when the membranes rupture prematurely labor may only occur 48 to 72 hours later. If there is a premature rupture, you will need to go into the hospital and have the fetal heart checked. If the heartbeat is normal, internal examination will be avoided, as it may introduce infection. Infection can be checked by testing your temperature every 4 hours, by doing a blood count from your arm twice daily, and by checking the fetal heart every 4 hours to see if it speeds up. If the baby's heartbeat remains normal, then you will wait for the spontaneous onset of contractions.

In some centers, amniocentesis is also used as a further check for infection. The amniotic fluid extracted is stained for the presence of bacteria. Lung maturity tests can also be done using this sample of fluid. This new approach to the use of amniocentesis for monitoring premature rupture of the membranes (before labor begins) is being evaluated still, but I am sure it will soon be an accepted part of treatment of this condition.

Why does the doctor sometimes artificially rupture the membranes during labor?

The membranes are ruptured by doing an internal examination and then catching the membranes with a plastic amniotomy hook. Since the membranes have no sensation the procedure is no more painful than cutting your nails. If the amniotic fluid is green or wine-colored, rather than clear or lemon-colored, it might be a sign of fetal distress. It might also be done to shorten labor; or to allow internal fetal monitoring should the need for it arise. To minimize the risk of prolapse of the umbilical cord, the rupture would only be performed if the baby's head was engaged.

3. *The show:* The passage of the show (the plug of mucus and blood in the cervix) is the third way labor may start, and it indicates that the cervix is dilated. Once this occurs, labor will either be under way or start within a few hours (usually between 5 and 8 hours). The size is a blob about the size of the palm of your hand. It is not uncommon to have a brown stain a few days before labor, or after an internal examination late in pregnancy, as a little of the show is released or disturbed by the cervix shortening or by the manual examination.

How do you deal with pain in labor?

With an enlightened attitude shared by you and your husband, and with confidence in yourself encouraged by your doctor and by prenatal classes, you may, as many women do, go through natural labor without analgesics or any trouble. However, I do feel that today there is sometimes too much emphasis put on women being able to perform "natural" labor, which results in making those who resort to the use of analgesics or an epidural anesthetic feel guilty or disappointed.

You must not feel a failure if you resort to the help of a pain reliever in labor. Epidural anesthesia (see pages 261–265) offers you a largely pain-free labor and delivery, with minimal risk to mother and baby, and it enables you to remain alert and "undrugged."

What causes premature labor?

It is important to understand that today, when we talk about prematurity we mean "immature"; that is, the pregnancy has not progressed beyond the thirty-sixth week, when the baby's lungs would be fully mature. We no longer consider a baby born weighing under 5½ pounds to be premature, as some babies born between 38 and 40 weeks weigh that amount. Length of gestation, not fetal weight, is now known to be the important factor in determining prematurity.

There are as many as 20,000 premature births a year in America. Why does it happen? Just as we don't know why labor starts at term, so we do not know why certain women go into premature labor. We do know some possible contributing causes, such as smoking, alcohol, poor nutrition; and certain geographic areas such as the South as well as the very high altitudes in the north and northwest of America also seem to have a higher incidence of premature births. Then there are obstetrical reasons such as urinary infections, hemorrhage either from placenta previa or placental separation, multiple pregnancy, or amnionitis (an infection that may be caused by a virus or bacteria in the fluid surrounding the baby). This last reason probably accounts for most cases where the cause of premature labor is given as unknown. Studies are now being conducted into the role of bacterial and viral infections, and medical journals have recently carried articles implicating a wide variety of bacteria or viruses that might cause premature labor. No doubt we will soon be nearer the truth.

Can emotional stress be a cause of premature labor?

I know many women believe this, and often a woman who has gone into premature labor will tell me of some upset in her life, or some serious argument she had with her husband, saying, "That's what set it off." Again, we do not know if stress is really a cause but it does seem very likely. Fear, fright, anxiety, stimulate the nervous system and that may trigger hormonal reactions (see pages 147–148 on the probable causes of labor). For this same reason, many premature labors settle down if the woman is admitted to the hospital and made to rest in bed. We can often prevent premature delivery without the use of any treatment other than rest and reassurance.

Now, however, we do have an effective method of treating premature labor, as I have previously mentioned (see page 212). The use of beta-mimetic agents was introduced in the U.S. in late 1981. The first approved drug of this class is ritodrine. Before beta-mimetics were discovered, various methods had been tried to stop labor, including heavy sedation, bed rest, and even alcohol (we used to tell mothers to drink a cognac at night in an attempt to prevent the onset of premature labor). None of these methods of treatment was very safe for the baby, and all were largely ineffective.

Just how do beta-mimetics work? The uterus has nerve endings that relax the uterine muscle and prevent contractions. It was discovered that beta-mimetics reinforce that action and prevent further contractions. Unfortunately, they are not the final answer because, besides sedating the uterus, they act upon the mother's heart muscle and increase her pulse rate, giving some women flutterings in the chest that can be uncomfortable and frightening. These drugs must not be given if you have heart disease, and an EKG must be administered prior to receiving them.

What should you do if you go into premature labor?

First call your doctor and go straight to the hospital; bypass waiting in the admissions office and go immediately to the labor floor. You will be observed for about 30 minutes to see if you are truly in labor.

If it is considered applicable in your case, the drug ritodrine will be administered intravenously, for up to 12 hours. It usually has a very dramatic effect in stopping contractions. After the 12 hours you will be put on oral ritodrine, and usually after a hospital stay of 48 hours you will go home.

The oral medication will be continued for as long as your

doctor thinks necessary. Contrary to many expectations, when you come off the drug it is unlikely that you will go into labor again. We now know that the onset of labor is *reversible*. This drug, you will be interested to note, does not suppress labor but *stops* it. You then go back to normal pregnancy—which is one of its greatest merits. You are not being kept in an artificially drug-induced state while taking ritodrine—in which case the minute you stopped it, you would go straight into labor. Rather, the drug aids the body in getting back into balance. This is also why we know more research must be done into the viral or bacterial infections that might be the cause of premature labor. If labor activity were set off, say, by a virus in the amniotic fluid (amnionitis), then what may be happening when ritodrine is administered is that it helps *contain* the pregnancy for as long as the virus is there, but once the viral infection has left the body there is no further danger of premature labor.

Not all premature labor is treated successfully or is treated at all. Premature labor is the commonest cause of neonatal mortality in America today. Some surviving premature infants may have neurological or intellectual impairment.

However, as you can see below (pages 222–224) there has been a very dramatic increase in the survival rate of immature infants. It is very important, therefore, if you are at high risk for premature labor (for example, if you have had a previous premature birth or you have a multiple pregnancy) that you be treated at a center equipped to deal with immature infants in an intensive care nursery. If you do deliver prematurely, even after taking ritodrine, you will want to feel confident that the hospital can provide skilled treatment for your child.

What if you have to be delivered before the baby's lungs are mature?

If you are in premature labor that cannot be stopped, or if an immediate induction is thought necessary, how will your doctor know whether the baby's lungs are immature? First, an amniocentesis can easily and quickly be done (in some hospitals they are done routinely on all women in premature labor) to test for fetal lung maturity and for amnionitis. The results for lung maturity can be back in as soon as an hour, depending on the technique used.

Immature lungs in the fetus may cause respiratory problems for the infant, necessitating prolonged use of an incubator or stay in a high-risk nursery. If your doctor feels that labor cannot be stopped, that it should not be stopped, or that induction is necessary, you will have to be delivered quite quickly. However, before delivery, your doctor can decide if there is time to administer a drug to *you* that can help to mature the baby's lungs within 12 hours. It takes 12 hours for the baby's lungs to complete their maturation and the effect of this injection may even be enhanced with a repeat dose after 12 hours. The drug effect will last about a week—so the birth must take place before then.

By now you must be wondering what I mean by "lung immaturity," and how it can be cleared up in 12 hours if it is such a serious problem. Inside the uterus the baby's lungs have a pink waterproof lining called the hyaline membrane. Just before birth, in late pregnancy, certain changes occur in the fetus. Agents are produced naturally that scour away the pink lining so that when the baby is born, the surface of the lungs is exposed and air can pass through them, enabling the baby to breathe in the outside world. The drug used to mimic this effect is a corticosteroid (a member of the cortisone group of drugs). It seems to work either by getting rid of the hyaline membrane directly or by encouraging the natural agents to do their work earlier.

Obviously there has been concern over the possible side effects of the drug on babies after birth. But recent studies have shown that so far there have been no long-term consequences. We have seen no incidence of medical problems and no evidence of lower IQ in babies so treated. In fact, we now have special studies from a doctor in New Zealand who has determined that corticosteroids are best used on women between the thirtieth and thirty-second week of pregnancy and that there is a small reduction in their efficacy before the thirtieth week and after the thirty-second (by the thirty-second week, the incidence of lung immaturity is much lower anyway). Corticosteroids are now used in most medical centers. (This maturing effect is actually one of the positive side effects of ritodrine, which, as I have explained, is used to stop premature labor activity.)

Even without corticosteroids the survival rate of premature infants is quite high today. But the use of the drug before birth does help relieve the parents of the anxiety of leaving their baby in an incubator for several weeks, of not being able to hold the child, feed it, or take it home with them—and of all the possible disruptions to their family life and bonding to this new baby that can be the consequences.

Why is labor induced?

Patients often express concern when they learn their labor is to be induced, worrying that induction is not really necessary, and that it is robbing them of their right to a natural childbirth. I would like to set the picture straight and reassure you that induction of labor is a great asset in modern obstetrics provided it is done strictly for medical reasons.

Induction means artifically starting labor rather than awaiting its natural onset. If you are in doubt about why your doctor is suggesting induction of labor for you, ask for a detailed explanation that includes all the alternatives. There are maternal and fetal reasons.

Maternal reasons are pre-eclampsia, hypertension, diabetes, heart disease, and antepartum bleeding. Some *fetal reasons* are placental insufficiency (the baby is in danger because it is not

getting enough food and oxygen from the placenta) and prolonged pregnancies (over 42 weeks). Basically, if the uterine
environment is not healthy for the baby, it is better to bring
on birth immediately rather than risk the baby's life by leaving
it longer inside you.

In the 1950s and 1960s, when the drugs that enabled the
induction of labor first became available, they were frequently
misused for social convenience. For example, there were instances when they were administered because the doctor was
going away and wanted to get the birth over with, or he or she
preferred a patient to go into labor at 9 A.M. on Thursday rather
than over the weekend or at night. Women, too, sometimes
asked to be induced so the birth could fall on their husband's
birthday or for the tax year, or so the child would be the right
age for the school year! We no longer accept such grounds as
being a valid indication for induction.

When such inductions became fashionable, there was insufficient backup of modern technology such as ultrasound and
amniocentesis to establish fetal maturity, and many babies were
born too early with respiratory problems. The rate of caesarean
sections also rose, because one of the complications of induction is failure to go into labor.

Now, however, we do have the backup technology. Induction has become one of the important advances in modern obstetrics, if it is performed for medical reasons and if it is done
correctly.

How is an induction done?

An appointment is made for you to be admitted to the labor
floor at a certain time (it is unusual for a hospital to allow elective inductions on weekends or public holidays). Your husband
may be with you all the time. Once you are in your hospital
gown, the fetal heartbeat will be monitored for about 20 minutes, and then you will be given an enema. The enema appar-

ently makes the uterus more irritable and likely to contract. Then your doctor will rupture the membranes with the amniotomy hook. An intravenous infusion will be started in your arm and Pitocin (synthetic oxytocin) may be added after about 30 minutes to start contractions.

While the Pitocin is being given it must be controlled continually by an intravenous pump and continuous fetal heart rate monitoring. Your doctor must be in attendance at all times. Pitocin got a bad name over the years; if it is misused, the resulting contractions can be so strong and unyielding, they will cause distress to the baby by not allowing the uterus to relax sufficiently so that blood can flow through it.

If controlled correctly, however, induced labor should not be more painful or different from natural labor. Using Pitocin, your obstetrician or midwife will be able to get you to the stage where you are having a *normal* labor.

So do not worry unduly if your labor has to be induced, as it is being done either for your or the baby's well-being. You can still do your breathing and push the baby out naturally, if you prefer to have completely natural childbirth. If it does become too painful, you can always request an epidural anesthetic or some other form of pain relief.

TESTS FOR FETAL WELL-BEING

There are many ways to assess the health and condition of the fetus throughout pregnancy. I have already discussed the role of ultrasound during the three trimesters. Most important, of course, is your doctor's continued clinical judgment. At each of your visits he or she will listen to the baby's heart and feel your abdomen externally to see if the baby's growth and the height of your uterus correspond to your dates.

There are now some fascinating new tests that give your doctor a very accurate idea of just how your baby is doing. Some are only possible in the third trimester when we are dealing with a large, healthy, active baby.

Fetal movement chart

This chart, which is kept by the mother, is a relatively new development in modern obstetrics. It relies on the mother's awareness of her baby's normal movements and on her alerting the doctor to any significant change.

The basic point is that the baby's movements in the third trimester are the best expression of its well-being. If it is kicking and writhing and squiggling about—it is healthy and happy.

We know mothers may feel fetal movements from as early as 18 weeks, though in early pregnancy the average number of movements per week is low. The number increases until, between the twenty-ninth and thirty-eighth week, they are at their maximum. In the last 2 weeks of pregnancy, the movements may change from actual kicks to writhing, since the baby is so big in relation to the amount of amniotic fluid.

The number of daily movements made by the average healthy baby (reported by mothers) varies between 4 and 1,400. As you can see, there is no absolute number. Most vary between 32 and 100 movements per day. There is no significance in the absolute number you record; only a change is significant.

One interesting point about the mother's sensitivity to fetal movements is that she in fact only picks up half of the actual amount of movements. We have noticed this phenomenon during ultrasound. If I, as the sonographer, compare what I see the baby doing with what the mother is describing as feeling, the baby actually moves far more than she realizes. I can only suppose that when the baby does not hit up against the uterine wall, its movements are not felt by the mother.

DAILY FETAL MOVEMENTS RECORDING

Name: _____

Date: _____

	1	2	3	4	5	6	7	8	9	10	11	12	13	14	15	16	17	18	19	20	21	22	23	24	25	Total		
Time:																											× 8 =	
Time:																											× 8 =	
Time:																											× 8 =	

Daily Total =

Date: _____

	1	2	3	4	5	6	7	8	9	10	11	12	13	14	15	16	17	18	19	20	21	22	23	24	25	Total		
Time:																											× 8 =	
Time:																											× 8 =	
Time:																											× 8 =	

Daily Total =

Date: _____

	1	2	3	4	5	6	7	8	9	10	11	12	13	14	15	16	17	18	19	20	21	22	23	24	25	Total		
Time:																											× 8 =	
Time:																											× 8 =	
Time:																											× 8 =	

Daily Total =

Time: _____ × 8 = ___
Time: _____ × 8 = ___
Time: _____ × 8 = ___

Daily Total = ☐

Date: _____

	1	2	3	4	5	6	7	8	9	10	11	12	13	14	15	16	17	18	19	20	21	22	23	24	25	Total

Time: _____ × 8 = ___
Time: _____ × 8 = ___
Time: _____ × 8 = ___

Daily Total = ☐

Date: _____

	1	2	3	4	5	6	7	8	9	10	11	12	13	14	15	16	17	18	19	20	21	22	23	24	25	Total

Time: _____ × 8 = ___
Time: _____ × 8 = ___
Time: _____ × 8 = ___

Daily Total = ☐

Date: _____

	1	2	3	4	5	6	7	8	9	10	11	12	13	14	15	16	17	18	19	20	21	22	23	24	25	Total

Time: _____ × 8 = ___
Time: _____ × 8 = ___
Time: _____ × 8 = ___

Daily Total = ☐

An actual fetal movement chart that you may use, following the instructions at the foot of the chart, in collaboration with your doctor.

How is a fetal movement chart kept?

The chart is filled out by you, by selecting three convenient times a day when, for 30 minutes at each of those times, you chart the number of movements your baby is making. What is a movement? Anything you feel—writhing or kicking. You could choose, for example, 8:30 to 9:00 A.M., 5:30 to 6:00 P.M., and 10:00 to 10:30 P.M.—they must be regular times when you know you can relax. You will find the process very reassuring; by forcing yourself to concentrate on the movements, you will re-alize that the baby is indeed moving. The records you keep will enable your doctor to assess whether the activity is ade-quate. Now that you are in your last trimester, every time you visit your doctor you will be asked about fetal movements.

The chart will show you that the baby might move around more in the evening than in the day, and that for periods of, say, half an hour, there are no movements at all. We assume these periods are when the baby sleeps. These rest periods are not constant, for babies in the uterus do not take regular naps—that is why the chart must be maintained over three 30-minute periods a day.

There is no difference in the amount of movements related to the mother's age, to the number of previous children, or to race, but if you smoke, they may decrease. It is also possible that various stimuli such as noise, external light, touch, ultra-sound, and regular and high-frequency waves will stimulate more movement in the baby.

From the seventh month of pregnancy, you must be ready to report any change in fetal movements either to the doctor or to the hospital. You must do this without fail if there are only three or four movements, or none at all, over a 12-hour period. Your doctor will follow up by listening to the baby's heart or with an ultrasound scan.

As an example of how this can be of help to the doctor, there is the story of a patient of mine, who was very near term, and who called me after a weekend to say she had not felt the baby move for 24 hours! She had been unwilling to disturb me at home at the weekend. (I use her example to show first, that you should call your doctor even on a weekend, and second, that the delay of even 24 hours need not be catastrophic.) I checked her immediately and found that the baby was alive, but that the placenta was not functioning well. We did an immediate caesarean section and the baby was delivered healthy and fine. We were all very relieved that the outcome was happy. This case shows that *you* can be one of the most effective monitors of your baby's health.

Even if your baby's movements seem to have ceased altogether, I advise you not to panic for fear that your baby must already be dead. There are many ways your doctor can quickly test the actual well-being of the infant, leading to a quick decision whether to induce labor, do a caesarean section, or do nothing at all but await natural delivery.

Antepartum fetal heart rate monitoring (AFHR)

AFHR is a method that enables us to assess, even long before labor, whether the baby is being supplied with all the oxygen and food that it needs. This technique developed as an outgrowth of the electronic monitoring routinely done during labor. Once electronic monitoring had been in use for some years, and the effects of the stress of a contraction were seen on the baby and fully understood, then it was realized we could get immediate information in the same way at any time in the third trimester on how the baby was faring and how it would react to labor.

What is happening to the baby in the uterus that makes it possible for us to elicit this information? When the uterus contracts and the uterine muscle squeezes on the blood vessels in its walls, it cuts off the baby's supply of oxygen and food for those moments. If the placenta and uterus are healthy and the baby has therefore been getting enough oxygen and glucose all through the third trimester, then the effect of the contraction will not show in the baby's heartbeat and the baby will be perfectly able to take the deprivation of the contractions.

But, if either the placenta or baby are not healthy, we will see that the baby's heartbeat *drops* after the induced contraction. This is a sign of fetal distress. It does not mean that the baby is going to die immediately. It tells us, however, that prolonging the pregnancy might be harmful.

Maybe your reaction to all this is to exclaim that electronic monitoring of fetal distress is the kind of technological intervention that has taken childbirth away from the mother and put it into the hands of the (male) doctors, depriving you of your right to a natural experience, and leading to an increase in caesarean-section deliveries. I would like to take this opportunity to explain a few things, which I will also discuss in greater detail in the next chapter on the birth process (see page 243).

First, this type of reaction used to have some truth in it. When electronic fetal heart rate monitoring first came into use, the medical profession's lack of experience with the equipment and lack of skill in interpreting the messages therein did lead to some unnecessary caesarean sections and to some uncalled-for inductions of premature labor. The criticism leveled at the obstetrics world was in part correct. But today, with years of experience in interpreting the fetal heart patterns, we can now be so accurate in detection of fetal distress that it is actually *lessening* the number of caesarean sections performed.

I am sure you have already thought of the question: If the monitoring depends on watching fetal heart activity during a uterine contraction, how can it be done *before* labor? The following discussion of nonstress testing and of contraction stress testing will provide the answer.

Nonstress testing

We know that when the normal baby moves in the uterus its heart speeds up. Such a reaction to movement shows us that the baby is well at the time. We also know that if the baby moves today, it will be well and just as healthy for up to 3 to 4 days more. So, if your baby is moving, you and your doctor can feel confident about letting the pregnancy continue for at least half a week more.

If you are going for a nonstress test make sure you do not smoke, take any sedating drugs, or drink alcohol beforehand. Have something to eat, preferably sweet, as glucose in your bloodstream will wake the baby.

How is the nonstress test done? The patient comes to her doctor's office, or to the labor floor in the hospital, and lies comfortably on her side, usually on an examining couch or bed. She is linked to a monitor that picks up the fetal heart rate, and a recorder is placed on her abdomen. Each time she feels the baby move, she is asked to press a button.

With this kind of test, your doctor will be looking for an acceleration in the baby's heart rate associated with a fetal movement and will also note the number of movements. We call this "fetal reactivity." To complete the test, we require two or more fetal heart rate accelerations of at least 15 beats per minute, which should last 30 seconds, associated with a movement (indicated by your pressing the button) over a 20-minute period. There will be a tracing of the heart movements on the recorder for you and your doctor to see.

This method is called nonstress testing because it does not involve uterine contractions and the baby's movements are voluntary. The only problem with nonstress testing occurs when the baby does not want to make any movements at all at that particular time. Your doctor will probably ask you if you have been smoking cigarettes recently, or whether you have taken any sedative drugs (such as Valium).

Contraction stress testing (CST)

Contraction stress testing is a refinement of the nonstress testing technique. The basic procedure is the same, except that in this test your doctor intervenes to *stimulate* uterine activity. That does not mean we induce labor, but we do simulate contractions, just as you would have in early labor. You will be closely monitored and the fetal heart rate and contractions will be recorded (they are merely the tightenings of the uterus you are familiar with as Braxton Hicks contractions).

For a CST you have to come to the hospital labor floor for an intravenous infusion; it cannot be given in your doctor's office.

You lie on a bed, just as for the nonstress test, with a monitor and recording device attached to your abdomen to trace the fetal heart rate and contractions. An intravenous line will be attached to your arm, into which Pitocin will be injected to cause contractions. It may sound heartless to make you go through contractions before labor; but remember, such a test is only done if your doctor has some concern as to the baby's health, and usually it is only performed if the nonintervening "nonstress" test has produced results that are doubtful or suspicious.

Once you are experiencing three contractions every 10 minutes, you will be watched for the effect of the stimulated labor on the fetus. Contraction stress testing is very sensitive and it will give your doctor accurate information about the state of your baby.

The sign that all is well with your baby is that there is no drop in the baby's heart rate after a contraction. If it drops, then your doctor knows there is insufficient utero-placental reserve, and the supply of food and oxygen to the baby is inadequate. When the uterus contracts, cutting off the supply for those few seconds, there is not enough glucose stored in the

234

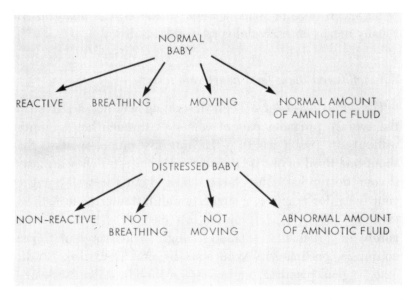

The chart shows how your doctor assesses 'bio-physical monitoring' from ultrasound in the third trimester (see page 237). Four simple points tell whether your baby is healthy and normal, or whether it is distressed.

baby's heart to maintain a healthy heartbeat right through the contraction and afterward.

How does your doctor decide which test to use?

Your doctor's decision on what must be done will be based on the following brief guidelines: if the nonstress test is normal, and the outlook for the rest of the pregnancy is excellent, the nonstress test will still be repeated weekly.

If the results of the first nonstress test prove abnormal, then you will have a contraction stress test. A CST result will reassure you and your doctor that everything is all right, since the CST is *very* accurate. Both the nonstress and the CSTs will be repeated once or twice a week. If the CST is abnormal, it usually means an early delivery is indicated.

Who will need these fetal heart rate tests?

The tests that I have been describing will *not* be given to the average pregnant patient who sails through her 9 months without any problems. In a teaching institution, we find that about one third of our patients have these tests. They are used if your doctor has cause for concern about the well-being of your baby (for example, a suggestion of intrauterine growth retardation [IUGR]), or if you fall into one of the high-risk categories of pregnancy (diabetes, high blood pressure, preeclampsia, postmaturity syndrome [beyond 42 weeks], Rh disease, vaginal bleeding, and other rare medical illnesses), or if you have been feeling diminished fetal movements, or have had an accident that might have injured you.

These are sophisticated new tests, and I must emphasize that they are not done in every doctor's office and hospital. If yours is a high-risk pregnancy, you should try to find a good obstetrician who is attached to a teaching hospital that has a neonatal intensive care unit. This could make all the difference to your pregnancy and to the health of your baby.

Why are fetal stress tests not part of routine pregnancy care?

Ideally, every woman should be monitored in this way late in the third trimester, so that we can all be confident that everything is happening for the best in each pregnancy. Obviously, this is impossible in terms of time, skilled manpower, and the financial burden of pregnancy. But it does mean we are entering a strange new phase now when, with the accurate assessment of high-risk patients and the exhaustive tests that are done on these women, the statistics are beginning to show up problems in the *low-risk* group. That is because, if anything serious does go wrong (and it rarely happens), the babies we may unfortunately lose belong to low-risk mothers in whom no one foresaw any problems. In fact, it now seems that over 70 percent of such sad instances take place with women who were not considered to be at high risk. Bearing that in mind, it does emphasize what I said earlier, about the value of keeping your own fetal movement chart, and remaining very aware of the pattern of your baby's movements throughout the third trimester.

Biophysical monitoring

Now I am going to describe to you a very new method of testing fetal well-being that has only been developed and put into practice within the last year. The use of ultrasound in the third trimester avoids the disadvantages of the contraction stress test (hospitalization, intravenous infusion, stimulation of contractions). So, if the nonstress test is abnormal, doctors seeking noninterventionist methods in obstetrics have begun to use this method next.

1. *Fetal breathing inside the uterus.* The motion of the baby's chest is watched for a period of 30 minutes. If the baby is seen to be breathing in this time, then that is a *splendid sign* that all is well. Recent work from California has even shown us that if your nonstress test has been abnormal but your doctor can *see* that your baby is breathing, then you can go home without any further tests or concern.

2. *The amount of amniotic fluid and its even distribution.* If there is fluid spread throughout the uterine cavity and it is at least 1 centimeter in depth, then you can be reassured that your baby is all right. (With intrauterine growth retardation, the amount of fluid is diminished.) This determination and the one above are most reliable.

3. *Fetal tone (how the baby flexes its limbs and returns to normal).* If the flexing is strong, this is a sign of a healthy baby.

237

Hormone tests in late pregnancy

Taking a sample of blood from your arm to test for the hormone *estriol* used to be a very popular test for fetal well-being. Estriol is an estrogen produced in great abundance during pregnancy, both by the fetus and the placenta. By measuring the amount of the hormone in your blood, it gives us an idea of how the placenta and the baby are faring. It is measured two or three times a week from the thirtieth week of pregnancy. One reading of estriol levels is of no use, as your doctor needs to see a continued upward rise over a length of time.

Some doctors do routine estriol testing, while others only administer the test for indications such as those described for prenatal monitoring. Estriol testing can be very helpful in cases of postmaturity (40+ weeks) if you have high blood pressure, Rh disease, a twin pregnancy, or if there is suspicion of IUGR.

We used to think estriol testing was very important. But now it is losing ground probably because the results are not immediately available (a few hours are required before the laboratory results can be obtained).

Moreover, we are aware that certain factors that do not relate to pregnancy can influence the hormone levels in the mother's blood, such as the time of day the test is done, or presence in the mother's system of aspirin or ampicillin.

Human placental lactogen (HPL) is another hormone that can be measured in late pregnancy, and testing for it is done in many centers. HPL is manufactured solely by the placenta during pregnancy and can also be measured in your blood. A normal and increasing level shows that your placenta is functioning properly.

Is there any way you can be sure your baby is all right?

There is at present no *single* prenatal monitoring test which on its own tells all about the baby. Rather, we have to rely on a consideration of all the tests that I have described in the preceding sections. Your obstetrician may prefer to run all or some of the tests if necessary and compare the results. Most important of all, you will have to rely on the skill and experience of your chosen doctor in interpreting information, and on his or her clinical judgment as to the actual state of your baby. With so much that can be done in late pregnancy to ensure the baby's safety, health, and well-being, these weeks should pass peacefully and without anxiety. Now you are about to enter into the particular birth process by which your baby will end its stay in the uterus and enter your arms.

THE MOTHER'S LIFE STYLE

Work

Most women will have come to their own conclusions by the third trimester as to their preferred way of living through this pregnancy. Experience has already shown us that working to term causes no problems for the average mother of a healthy baby. No one is going to stop you from *working* until the day you go into labor if you so wish. However, many employers recommend that a woman take maternity leave at least 3 to 4 weeks before she is due. I do not recall any stories of women giving birth on the office floor or in the elevator, so you need have no anxieties on that score. If there has been any medical reason for you to stop work, this will already have been suggested by your doctor. Sometimes stopping work a month before the birth can make you feel *so* much better that you wonder why you did not do it earlier. It's not a new idea, but I do recommend it.

Any incidence of high blood pressure, hypertension, or suggestion of IUGR (if your weight gain has been too slow) will have led to the advice that you give up work around the end of the second trimester. Tiredness is an obvious problem for those women who do work right to the end, but many working women feel it is better to put in all the hours they can now, so they can take as long as possible off work once the baby has been born. Obviously you should avoid overexertion. Travel to work and home in the most comfortable fashion, even arranging to leave work early to beat the rush hour. Get plenty of sleep. And get your feet off the floor for as many hours a day as possible.

Exercise

Whether you feel like continuing active or vigorous *exercise* now is up to you. Only you can judge how fit and energetic you feel and whether the activity of jogging, swimming, or some gentle exercise is leading to undue tiredness or excessive Braxton Hicks contractions. Your doctor will have advised against any further vigorous exercises if you have been suffering a lot of Braxton Hicks or have been feeling any low abdominal cramps. If you have had some spotting of blood and mucus (though not the show itself, which is large enough to fill the palm of your hand), you should probably give up vigorous exercises now as this spotting might indicate that labor is imminent. But many women I know have jogged right up to the day of labor. And even more women manage to fit in a swimming program right through the third trimester. If at all possible, continuing to exercise is healthy, and it is wonderful to begin the process of motherhood so fit and positive in your approach. Through whatever means, do try to keep physically fit.

Travel

Distant travel is contraindicated in the third trimester. However, if you are on a car trip about an hour's journey away from home, do not panic if early labor contractions should begin.

This stage will go on for several hours, giving you ample time to return and to get to the hospital.

Before making travel plans that will cross into the late third trimester, check with your airline or cruise ship for their policy on travel in late pregnancy. Most airlines limit their carriage to women no closer than 4 weeks from their due date.

Large cruise ships, such as the *Queen Elizabeth 2* do carry a small and limited medical staff, but you will have to sign a disclaimer of their responsibility should you give birth on board. Such ships have a doctor on board who can manage a normal pregnancy. But the physician may not be capable of performing a caesarean section, and the ship is certainly not equipped for neonatal intensive care, should the baby need treatment.

A friend of mine who was 33 weeks pregnant traveled on the *Queen Elizabeth 2*, danced in the ship's discos, jogged around the deck, and took part in on-board yoga classes. She described it as a wonderful experience, even if fellow passengers did regard her as somewhat crazy. She only admits to fears after the event, when her baby was delivered by her doctor here in New York, by caesarean section as it happened (because she suddenly started to lose blood vaginally from placental separation), just 3 weeks after docking. She hates now to think what might have happened to her on board. Sometimes, at the beginning of the third trimester, it is hard to believe that your baby will come early, or that you could go into premature labor.

Do listen to your doctor's advice on the subject of travel. He or she will know whether you should remain near your home and hospital. None of the sophisticated monitoring methods I have described in previous sections is available either 3,000 feet up in the sky or 300 miles out at sea.

Sex

You should be able to have sex any time in pregnancy, till you go into labor. In fact, some couples use sexual intercourse as a way of encouraging labor to come on if the baby is late. Intercourse may promote the onset of labor because, as I have previously explained, male semen contains prostaglandin, the hormone that helps set off uterine contractions.

But if sex can be used to bring on a late baby, is it safe to have intercourse in late pregnancy? The answer is difficult to define, but I can only say that we do not know exactly what makes labor start, but we do know that prostaglandin, ejaculated into the vagina as part of your husband's semen, will not set off labor contractions if your baby is not ready to be born.

If your doctor has noticed that the membranes are showing or that your cervix has begun to dilate, you will be advised to stop sexual intercourse for fear of introducing infection. You can of course continue other forms of sexual activity. Or, you might prefer to indulge in massage, caresses, being loving and excited together about the birth. Please be assured, though, that most couples do manage to have sex, without fear, throughout the third trimester.

CHAPTER

5

Labor

Many women pregnant for the first time can imagine labor and looking after the baby, but they find it hard to imagine what comes in between. To help dispel the aura of mystery that surrounds birth itself, I will address myself here to the sorts of questions women ask to relieve some of the tension. I will also explain all the most up-to-date methods we have for watching the health of your baby throughout the labor and delivery process.

What causes labor to start?

It is amazing, in light of all the advancements that have been made in obstetrics and the kinds of technology we have developed, that we do not know exactly what causes a woman to go into labor. Our knowledge is increasing, however, and current research work is showing that it is probably not due to one mechanism alone, but to a combination of factors. A shift in your hormonal pattern, caused by an increase in oxytocin, is an important—but not the single—factor in setting off labor. Other hormones, such as the recently discovered prostaglandins, play a very important part, as do estrogen and progesterone in the bloodstream.

It is also likely that the fetus helps dictate when contractions begin, because certain changes in the baby's adrenal glands favor the release of prostaglandins in the uterus, which, combined with oxytocin, will make contractions begin. So if you have been fantasizing that your baby has a mind of its own and decides when to "come out," you may not be so far wrong!

This complex interaction of hormones is sometimes called the "see-saw" theory. For example, if the level of progesterone drops, that will allow hormones like oxytocin and prostaglandin to rise. It also explains why we can *stop* premature labor activity with drugs, or bed rest, as I have previously described. The drug ritodrine allows the hormones to assume their normal balance. The significant role of the fetus in dictating when labor begins also emphasizes why it can be very dangerous to stop the labor activity in certain cases of prematurity.

According to one theory, when the uterus and baby reach a certain size, there is less amniotic fluid present and so more contact between the baby and the walls of the uterus; this in itself may contribute to the onset of contractions.

Can you encourage labor to start?

As I mentioned at the end of the previous chapter, your doctor will be on the lookout for any problem with your baby if you go beyond your due date. Otherwise, leave the delivery date to nature.

What will happen when you come to the hospital?

If labor has begun, it is a good idea not to eat or drink anything. Even if you are going to have natural childbirth, you never know if you might need an emergency caesarean. The presence of food and drink, in the stomach, may lead to problems with anesthesia.

I will not build up your expectations of what will happen when you arrive at the hospital. Although you might secretly desire a warm and pleasant place, with tasteful decor and the comforts of home, and although some hospitals have indeed improved their obstetrics accommodations to create this effect, many modern teaching hospitals are frankly run-down and quite seedy-looking. Medical centers in large urban areas deal with every emergency, and they show it! Whatever your esthetics, the important thing is to be in a place where you know that excellent care and every modern technique are available.

On entering the hospital, go straight to the labor floor. Do not stop at admissions (you might still be there when you give birth). Women in labor, as in any emergency, may bypass admissions. Your husband can go along there later to give the necessary information.

At the Mount Sinai Hospital, for example, when you come in suspecting you are in labor, you go straight to a bed on the labor floor. You get changed and a monitor is put on your abdomen. If your doctor is not already there, a resident will monitor your contractions, check the fetal heart rate, and give you a vaginal examination to determine whether labor has actually begun. The resident is not there to substitute for your own doctor, who will be on hand for most of the labor process as well as the delivery.

Will you be shaved? Surprisingly, this is now quite a controversial topic. Personally, I do not encourage shaving, because the evidence seems to point to the fact that shaving encourages infection, rather than discouraging it, which was the whole point of the procedure in the first place. Your doctor may order a little perineal shaving (between the vagina and the anus), as that is the only place hair can get in the way. If your hair is very long on the labia, it might be difficult to stitch up an epi-siotomy. But it is unnecessary to go through the whole ritual for every birth.

Should you give yourself an enema before coming into the hospital? You may be more comfortable doing it at home than being given an enema in the hospital. (You can buy the dispos-able Fleet enemas for this purpose.) Even if you have had a bowel movement recently, it would not have emptied the lower rectum of all material, and a full rectum may delay labor.

From this point on, the management of your pregnancy will depend on your obstetrician. Your temperature and pulse will be recorded and your urine will be tested. A blood sample will be taken from your arm to determine your blood status and in case it needs to be cross-matched for a transfusion. If your la-bor is not too far advanced, a resident will come to take your history for the hospital chart.

What is the difference between a birthing room and a labor room?

Most of the major teaching hospitals now have a birthing room available for those who request it (providing the demand does not exceed availability on the day you go into labor). The birthing room is meant to be unclinical, more like home than a hospital. It contains a birthing bed, which is different from the average labor bed as it alters posture in many different ways and can come apart to act as a delivery table too. Al-though the birthing bed is technically sophisticated, it is dis-guised to resemble your bed at home. The birthing room will be furnished with easy chairs for your husband, a TV, a phone, and a refrigerator where you can store champagne to greet the birth. These rooms are not prepared for any specialized medi-cal procedures, so if you need anything like epidural anesthesia or intravenous Pitocin, you will have to be moved to a regular

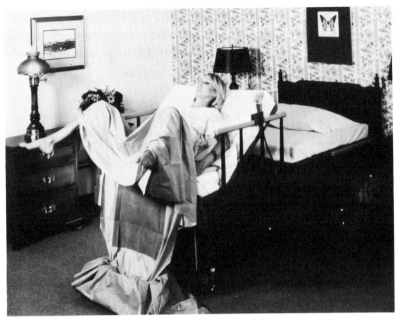

The birthing bed and a typical birthing room setting. For delivery, the bed divides and the baby will be born in this pleasant environment without your being taken to a delivery room.
Courtesy of B–W Health Products™.

labor room. But that need not be so bad. You can still get a single labor room and have your husband with you.

Even if you are in a labor room, you can have natural childbirth. You stay there for the first stage of labor and, once fully dilated, you will be moved into a delivery room, which is a modified operating room.

If you labor in a birthing room, you deliver the baby there too.

LABOR

Labor is divided into three stages. The first stage is from the onset of labor activity until full dilation of the cervix, that is,

10 centimeters, has been reached. The second stage is involved with the delivery (sometimes the rather insensitive word *expulsion* is used) of the baby, and the third stage is the interval from the birth to the expulsion of the placenta.

What will happen to you during labor?

Early labor activity should be spent at home. Once in the hospital I'd advise you to walk about. Today most labor floors will permit you to walk, as it has been shown in many studies that walking encourages the progress of labor, perhaps because it helps your body to work with gravity rather than against it. It will also make early labor less boring and more comfortable for you.

What is the progression of labor through the three stages?

The first stage covers the whole of the first portion of labor, from the mild contractions of early labor when your cervix is effacing (shortening) and beginning to dilate, through the stronger and more established contractions until full dilation takes place. Half of the time of labor may be involved with effacement, so there is ordinarily no rush in getting to the hospital once contractions begin. Emanuel Freedman, from Harvard, has worked out a curve to show the expected changes in the opening of the cervix. The initial contractions begin effacement; then dilation starts slowly, and by the time the cervix is 2 or 3 centimeters dilated, effacement is usually complete. Once at that point, since the cervix already has no length, dilation from 3 to 8 centimeters is very rapid. In this acceleratory phase you will be dilating 1.1 to 1.5 centimeters an hour. Then the rate halves again for the last phase of dilation, from 8 to 10 centimeters, and the contractions slow down and change in character.

I have explained this curve to you for a reason. Less so that you should be aware of the level of pain and contractions to expect at each stage (your Lamaze classes will have taught you that), than to explain what is happening each time your obstetrician or midwife examines you. The purpose of the vaginal examination is not only to see how far you have already progressed but to check how far, in the examiner's mind, you *should* have progressed. For example, if at 2 P.M. you are 4 centimeters dilated, then your doctor knows that by 5 P.M. you should be almost 7 centimeters dilated. If you are not, then he or she will want to know *why*. In this way, we ensure that labor progresses normally. In Britain, they use what is known as a *partogram*, where a record is kept of these findings in each labor and compared to a curve similar to the one described above. If certain lines cross the curve, then that alerts the physician to the fact you are not progressing as you should be.

In early labor, the intrauterine pressure is low and your contractions will be short. As labor progresses, contractions will last longer, about 40 to 45 seconds, and as pressure within the uterus rises, some discomfort is felt. Once you cannot breathe through your contractions, then you should be on your way to the hospital.

The best position for the baby in terms of your own comfort during labor is when it is lying head down on its abdomen, hugging your spine. When you feel contractions in your back, rather than in the lower abdomen, it is known as back labor, and it means that the baby is probably lying in the correct position (head down), but it is on its back, looking upward, as if sunning itself. This posterior position can make labor more uncomfortable for you and can add up to 2 hours to the length of your labor. In the old days, before there were adequate forms of pain relief, such a labor could sometimes drive a woman to say afterward, "never again." However, the discomfort of back labor can now be treated with an epidural anesthetic, and Pitocin given intravenously will improve the quality of your contractions and encourage the baby to move its head from a

posterior to an anterior position. Back labor is usually a problem of first pregnancies and may not recur.

Intrauterine pressure and the discomforts of contractions are
greatest toward the end of the first stage. Your breathing and
preparation will be especially useful now. You may ask for some
form of pain relief if you feel the need. The first stage will
usually last under 12 hours (less for second and subsequent
children).

Some women have very rapid labor, lasting only 1 or 2 hours,
which we call precipitate labor. And others have lengthy labor,
sometimes over 24 hours, which we call prolonged labor. Fortunately we are seeing less of prolonged labor as preparation
for childbirth has reduced tension (which led to poor-quality
contractions). Better understanding of the normal working of
labor has also led to improvement, as have better nourishment,
better social conditions, and the fact that although women now
have bigger babies they also tend to have bigger pelves (see
page 213).

As you go into the second stage (at full dilation), you will
notice the transition yourself. It may be heralded by vomiting
or shivering, but the most obvious clue is the nature of the
contractions, because, although they are stronger than ever and
the pain is at a maximum, there is a desire to bear down because of the pressure of the baby's head (which has descended
farther) on your rectum. Remember, too, that the membranes,
unless previously broken, may rupture at this point.

Full dilation is confirmed by your doctor's examination to see
that the cervix has disappeared. You will be encouraged by the
nurse, or midwife, to push *with* contractions, as your pushing
and the uterine contractions help move the baby down through
the pelvis. Soon the top of the scalp can be seen through the
distended vaginal opening. This slow appearance of the head is
called "crowning." It is a very exciting moment. Your husband
will be able to watch the whole event until you, with the help
of a suitably angled mirror, will also be able to see the crown-

ing. If you are in a birthing room, you will deliver there; or, if you are on the labor floor, you will be moved to the delivery room.

The second stage is involved with the delivery of the baby (for more detailed description of the various methods of delivery, see pages 267–280). The second stage may last up to an hour in a woman who has previous children, or up to 2 hours for a first baby. Your doctor is not likely to intervene unless a problem arises.

At the end of the second stage, as the head releases from your vagina, an episiotomy may be performed (see pages 268–269). An episiotomy is an incision into the lower part of the vagina and perineum (the area between the vagina and anus) to widen the birth outlet. It will not be done routinely, but for various indications to prevent the tearing of vaginal tissue and subsequent scar formation (which could later lead to painful intercourse). Moreover, if the vaginal tissue is overstretched, it could lead to a prolapse weakening of tissues later in life that can be very discomforting.

The period after the baby has been born is known as the third stage. The umbilical cord is clamped and cut. (Your husband may cut the cord if he desires.) The baby is given to you and your husband. You may even put the baby to the breast. You now have to wait for the placenta to be expelled, but this should be a comfortable and relaxed time for you. It can last for as little as a few minutes or as long as an hour, averaging about 5 to 10 minutes.

Once the placenta has been expelled, you may be given some Pitocin by intravenous or intramuscular injection to keep the uterus contracted. (If the uterus were to relax that could lead to bleeding.) Pitocin is specifically given to mothers of twins, to women who have had excessive bleeding in a previous pregnancy, or who are having a fifth or subsequent pregnancy.

The baby will then be taken from you and placed in a warmer, where a pediatrician will check the infant thoroughly, and a nurse will place antibiotic ointment into its eyes to prevent any possibility of gonococcus infection. The baby will be supplied with identification in the form of wrist bands bearing your name, and two bare footprints and thumb prints will be taken—all of which information is recorded so there is no room for mistakes.

While this is going on, your blood pressure and pulse will be checked. You may experience shivering or feel nauseated. Though it is not quite clear why you can have such symptoms, they may be due to absorption by your body of some of the amniotic fluid.

Your doctor will repair the episiotomy if one was done. If you are in the delivery room (not the birthing room), your baby will then be handed back to you, and you will be taken to the recovery room for a few hours. Your baby will spend some 30 minutes with you in the recovery room and will then be taken to the nursery to be weighed (for the first time) and kept warm. Meanwhile, you will be observed for about 2 to 3 hours, and then you will be wheeled to your bed in the maternity unit to await your baby's return.

What is your doctor watching for during labor?

Your doctor wants to ensure that labor progresses and that you will remain well and not develop any symptoms of *maternal distress*. The symptoms of maternal distress are dehydration, high fever, and exhaustion. Fortunately, this condition rarely occurs today because it can be prevented, even long before pregnancy begins, by better general health care. Once you are pregnant, it is guarded against with good prenatal care, advice about nutrition, and by sympathetic medical treatment providing both explanation and understanding of childbirth.

Apart from maternal stress, the most important factor watched for is any sign of *fetal distress*. Since maternal mortality in childbirth has become extremely rare, the last few years have enabled us to turn our energies toward a different sphere of obstetrics: the health and safety of the fetus.

How can fetal distress be monitored?

In the last few years, we have come to rely heavily on electronic fetal monitoring during labor. Fetal monitors produce a tracing of the peaks and valleys of your contractions and of the baby's heart rate. We know that there are safe and normal patterns of the baby's heart rate (see pages 254–257) during and after a contraction, and your doctor will watch for these patterns at all times during labor.

Even though you are likely to keep your eyes glued to the monitor, please bear in mind that the majority of alterations in the recorded pattern do not mean the baby is distressed or in danger, or that you will have to have a caesarean section. The interpretation of the monitor pattern requires skill and experience in the physiology of contractions and fetal response.

Before electronic fetal monitoring became available, the traditional way of monitoring fetal well-being was for the midwife or doctor to listen to the baby's heartbeat with a stethoscope, and at the same time to keep a hand on the mother's abdomen to detect the beginning and end of a contraction. This procedure was done only intermittently, and the new machines have enabled us to improve upon and simplify a repetitious task.

There has been a lot of controversy lately over whether the use of the electronic fetal monitors has led to a dramatic increase in the rate of caesarean sections. The rate may indeed have gone up initially, but now experience with monitoring and more sophisticated machines has actually increased our understanding of the different fetal heart patterns and the reasons for them, so, in fact, monitoring has *reduced* the overall caesarean-section rate in very recent times.

External monitoring

External electronic fetal monitors are used in the following way. During labor, a small machine called a cardiotochograph stands next to your bedside, and a clover-leaf fetal heart rate detector and a small box, a contraction detector, are strapped to your abdomen. The machine, which is very sensitive, records on paper a continuous heart rate and contraction pattern for you and the doctor to see. We can tell extremely early on if anything is beginning to go wrong and whether it is necessary to take any alternative measures, about which you will read more as this chapter continues.

During a normal contraction, the blood supply to the baby and to the placenta is cut off for a number of seconds. This will not harm your baby at all, providing the placenta is operating properly. The fetal heart rate should either remain unaltered or drop slightly during the contraction. This kind of fetal heart rate drop is recorded on the monitor as the normal pattern that we call a "Type I dip."

One classical sign of fetal distress is if the drop in the heart rate comes *after* a contraction (Type II dip) and the drop takes a long time to return to normal. This is regarded as an abnormal pattern. But an abnormal pattern alone no longer calls for a red alert. These changes *precede* any acid base (chemical) alterations in the baby that might do harm. Since the monitor can detect these changes very early on, the distress can often be remedied. Your doctor will check to see why the pattern is going this way. You may be put on your side to see if a change of position will alter the pattern, or you may be given oxygen. As a double check on the baby's well-being, your doctor can take a fetal scalp blood sample (see below, pages 257–259). These reassuring steps work toward preventing the necessity of a caesarean section.

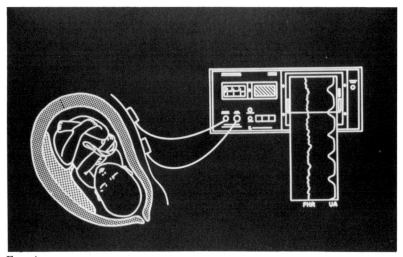

Fig. A.

Fig. B.

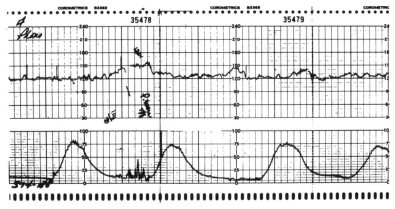

FIG. A. The fetal monitor attached to your abdomen traces the pressure of the mother's contraction and the pattern of the fetal heartbeat before, during, and after a contraction.

FIG. B. The top line shows the normal pattern of a contraction and the bottom line shows the fetal heartbeat reaction to that pressure.

Yale University Medical School, Dept. of Ob/Gyn, Perinatal Unit.

Internal monitoring

An even more sophisticated form of fetal heart rate monitoring is known as "internal monitoring." If the fetal heart rate signal is not recording well on the external clover-leaf lead because of disturbance being picked up from your own heartbeat, or if the machine keeps losing the beep owing to your movements as you change positions, we can use an internal monitor. Instead of placing the clover-leaf heart rate detector on your abdomen, a lead is taken from the cardiotochograph machine through your vagina and cervix, and an electrode at the end is attached to the baby's scalp. The electrode gives a direct reading that is very accurate, and that can be of great advantage in some circumstances. But how, you must be wondering, can a lead from the monitor be attached to your baby's scalp during labor? Do not be alarmed by the sound of this procedure. No one is going to drill a hole in the baby's head! We advisedly use the word *scalp*, as the electrode is attached by a little coiled needle to a tiny piece of skin on the baby's head. This skin has few nerves or blood vessels, and the procedure will not hurt your baby, nor will it cause any damage to the baby's head or hair growth. It is quite comfortable for you; it is a sterile procedure performed during an internal examination. The cervix must be at least 3 to 4 centimeters dilated before the electrode can be put in position.

Internal monitoring of the uterine contractions (pressure) can also be done by using a fluid-filled catheter that would also be inserted through the vagina and cervix. But we seldom use this procedure, mainly because it carries a risk of infection.

A fetal monitor can easily be detached so you can walk around the room. And, if you wish, monitoring can be done intermittently rather than continuously. The external monitor can be used in the birthing room and does not in any way discourage natural childbirth. In fact, if anything, it helps encourage natural childbirth, since it enables your doctor to be confident about letting your labor progress to its natural end.

Still another great advantage is that monitoring techniques require constant supervision of the mother (as well as the baby), and this in itself is beneficial to labor. It is certainly better than being left alone in a room to scream your way through, as was once common practice.

Why and how does your doctor take a sample of fetal blood?

In the above discussion of internal monitoring, I described how an electrode can be attached to your baby's scalp during labor. In the same way, unbelievable though it may seem, before the baby is born we can take a few drops of blood from its scalp. From that sample, a very accurate assessment can be made, quickly and easily, that will tell us about the baby's *actual* state of well-being.

If the baby is suffering any degree of distress through lack of oxygen (if the placenta is not working properly), then the acid levels in its blood will be high. When a scalp sample has been taken, these levels can easily be read on a machine as a low or a normal pH. Very low pH (an indication of acid build-up in the baby's blood) indicates that the baby should be promptly delivered.

Fetal scalp blood sampling is done with utmost care and sensitivity and requires special training. The technique was introduced about 10 years ago by Dr. Fred Saling in Germany. It does not harm or traumatize the baby and has been of enormous benefit to obstetrics.

When would a fetal blood sampling be done? If the fetal heart rate patterns continue to be abnormal on the monitor, then the fetal blood sample can be repeated, checking the baby's blood acid levels as often as every *half hour* if necessary, until normal delivery is achieved; if these continue to show acidity (low pH), then the baby must be delivered promptly.

This procedure serves as a very active safeguard against *unnecessary* caesarean section, as, if your baby's heart rate *appears* abnormal, but the blood sample shows normality, then you can rest at ease that all is well and natural labor may be allowed to progress.

Bearing in mind the current medico-legal climate, it is important to remember that if your doctor sees an abnormal pattern on the monitor, he or she is duty-bound to make some sort of quick decision about delivery of your baby. Failure to react to the monitor reading could lead not only to some harm coming to your baby, but to the doctor's being sued for negligence.

How is fetal scalp blood sampling performed?

Your legs will be held in stirrups as for delivery. The vagina is cleansed and then an endoscope (a conical metal tube) is passed through the vagina and cervix to the fetal head. It looks in fact like a small ice cream cone with the end bitten off. It is illuminated by a light source at its entrance. The doctor wipes the baby's scalp and sprays it with a local anesthetic. A tiny blade on a long handle is passed through the endoscope, which has lit up the scalp area, and it pricks only the scalp skin. The doctor collects a few drops of blood in a fine glass tube, draws it out of the endoscope, and passes it to an assistant. The blood is put into a pH meter and the values are read off automatically by the machine. If the level is over 7.25, all is well and labor may progress. If the level is under that figure, then repeat fetal blood samples are necessary. If the level drops below 7.20, then your doctor will know to deliver you as rapidly as possible.

Fetal blood scalp sampling can only be done once you are in labor, and at least 3 to 4 centimeters dilated, sufficient to allow the endoscope through the cervix. The entire procedure takes in all about 5 minutes, and the results can be read in 1 minute.

Because this is such a sensitive method and the information it gives is so valuable, a new technique is being developed that will allow continuous pH readings, rather the way internal monitoring gives continuous fetal heart rate recordings. An electrode acting as a pH monitor would be attached to the baby's scalp. We have not yet been able to develop an electrode small enough to make this technique acceptable, but it is a development of the future to be watched for.

Are there any risks involved with fetal blood sampling?

There have been recent studies into the risk of infection in the puncture wound on the baby's scalp. Fortunately, it seems to be a very rare complication, and even that risk can be minimized by good technique and strict cleansing of the vagina and fetal scalp. The risk of bleeding from the puncture site in the scalp is negligible.

In most surveys that have been performed at the large teaching hospitals in the U.S., the evidence seems conclusive that fetal heart rate monitoring and fetal blood sampling are *very* beneficial. We are now seeing, for example, far fewer babies who are born with low levels of alertness, and we lose far fewer babies than we used to. The "good old days" were *not* so good in terms of perinatal mortality or morbidity.

PAIN RELIEF

Should you accept pain-relieving drugs during labor?

Because of some recent controversies over the idea of giving women any form of pain relief during labor, you may wonder why it is allowed and whether there is any danger involved in taking such drugs.

Let me first say that no one today should force pain relief on you. If you have been to prenatal classes, the fear and tension that can help promote pain in labor should be diminished. You will have a better understanding of what to expect, and how to control or bear the level of pain. I have watched many women in recent years positively sail through labor.

At the same time, let me add that I do not think you should suffer unduly and then afterward blame your obstetrician. You should go through labor to see what you can achieve, not what you can endure. If you feel the need for pain relief, despite your attempts at correct breathing and relaxation, it should be provided on request. So that brings us to the question of what forms of pain relief are available and whether they are proved safe.

Analgesics

Most medical centers will offer you the choice of analgesics or regional anesthesia (see pages 261–262). Adequate pain relief can often be achieved by the use of a narcotic such as Demerol, which is the most popular drug given to women in labor. It is given by injection either intravenously or intramuscularly. It is *very* effective as a pain reliever, though too high a dosage may mean that the mother goes through labor and delivery in a sedated cloud, unaware of the event. Demerol also has the disadvantage of crossing the placenta and sedating the fetus. This will not cause long-term harm, but it can mean that the baby will be born slightly depressed, in which case a reversant drug will be used to counter the effect of the Demerol.

The effect of the Demerol can be reversed before delivery (especially if the drug was administered less than 2 hours before). The mother is given an antagonizer to the narcotic, such as niloxone, so that she and the baby will both be awake for this important event. Both Demerol and its antagonist have been proved safe, and no complications other than that mentioned have been recorded. Promethazine hydrochloride can be added to Demerol to enhance its effect, and it is most often used today in a small dose, late in labor, if there is not enough time for an epidural to take effect before delivery.

If you read any older prenatal care books, you may see a much longer list of agents mentioned, classifying them into sedatives, analgesics, and inhalants. But few of these are used in the U.S. today. We have narrowed our field of options down to the agents we know are both effective and safe. The most common and popular form of pain relief now asked for, and given, is a regional anesthetic known as an epidural.

Epidural anesthesia

Epidural anesthesia, in which only the lower part of your body is anesthetized, has made a vast difference in the management of discomfort during labor. We know that the pain-carrying nerves from the uterus and the cervix pass through the lower spine, and it is at this point that an epidural anesthetic is put to work.

For an epidural, no needle or anesthetic agent enters the spinal canal itself. The vertebral column (spine) is constructed in a very fortunate way, because there is an area outside the spinal cord and its surrounding fluid into which the anesthetic can be inserted.

If your epidural anesthetic is well given, you should be able to move your legs quite satisfactorily while the anesthetic lasts, although they may feel heavy. Do not panic, however, having read this, if you cannot move your legs during your epidural. It does not mean something dreadful has happened and you will be paralyzed. The effect will wear off within a fairly short space of time after delivery: maybe half an hour, depending on the dose.

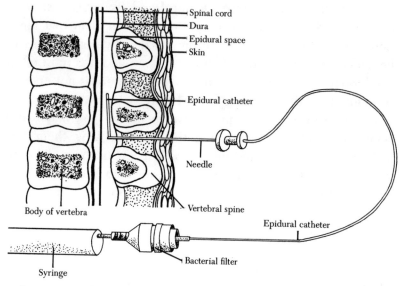

Spinal cord
Dura
Epidural space
Skin

Epidural catheter

Needle

Body of vertebra

Vertebral spine

Epidural catheter

Bacterial filter

Syringe

Where an epidural is given. The needle giving the anesthetic goes through your back into the epidural space, and *not* into the spinal cord.

When will you be given an epidural?

As the purpose of the epidural is pain relief and the effect is universally felt to be wonderful, it will be given when your obstetrician, and you yourself, feel that the discomfort of labor is great enough to require help. Other than having no medication at all, you will find an epidural the most natural form of pain relief. As the anesthetic is local, it does not affect the baby, who will be born completely "undrugged." You will remain wide awake; you may talk to your doctor, husband, or nurse, or just sit back and read a magazine if you wish. You can rest assured that there will be no side effects to your baby. He or she will come out very alert.

Another virtue of the epidural is that it can be given at any time during labor. You do not have to be dilated a certain degree. But, remember, it requires 20 minutes to take its full analgesic effect, so you might be advised to request it before the pain becomes too much to bear.

Certain conditions positively favor epidural anesthesia. For example, if the baby is not receiving a full placental blood supply (placental insufficiency) or if the mother is suffering from hypertension or pre-eclampsia. Also, epidural anesthesia is now used regularly for caesarean section. In fact, 75 percent of the caesarean sections performed in the past 6 months at Mount Sinai Hospital were done under regional rather than general anesthetic.

The commonest condition demanding the use of regional anesthetic is what we call "incoordinate labor." In this situation, the mother is very likely having her first baby, which is lying head down as it should be but in a "posterior presentation": its head is facing up at the ceiling. The mother will usually be progressing poorly in labor. Her contractions will be intense, and, in this condition, she might have to spend hours in labor. (In the old days, this was the kind of labor that went on for 20 hours.) We used to call the condition the Terrible Triad—first baby, posterior position, and incoordinate labor. In the end, it often led to symptoms of maternal distress from the painful, long labor and, therefore, to an emergency caesarean section.

This condition can now be corrected with an epidural anesthetic. We do not know why it has such a dramatic effect, but it is accompanied with relief all around. The mother's labor becomes normal and she begins to make good progress. She is able to deliver naturally and without caesarean section.

Who should not have an epidural?

Epidural anesthetic is contraindicated in certain instances. It cannot be used if you are about to deliver, as it takes 20 minutes to take full effect, and you might end up being delivered before the anesthesia has worked. It cannot be given if you are allergic to local anesthetics or if you have had a spinal injury or operation. If you are trying for a vaginal delivery after a previous caesarean section (see pages 276–277), you will not be allowed to have this form of pain relief, as it may mask symptoms of the scar rupturing. You should take note, too, that an anesthetist will be reluctant to give you an epidural if you have a history of back pain, as, if you think the epidural has subsequently aggravated the back pain, you might be inclined to lay medico-legal blame at the anesthetist's door after the delivery.

Who will give the epidural anesthetic?

Epidural anesthesia requires skill and experience in administration. It should only be given by an anesthetist skilled in the technique, and never by someone who has not been trained in its administration or who gives them infrequently. At Mount Sinai Hospital, for example, we have an attending obstetrical anesthetist on the labor floor 24 hours a day (not the same one, I hasten to add) who is an expert in the technique. But, if you deliver in a smaller hospital, you may find that no anesthetist qualified to administer an epidural is readily available.

How is an epidural given?

First, an intravenous line is started to keep you hydrated, in case of a fall in blood pressure. The insertion of the epidural anesthetic is a sterile technique, so your back will be cleaned, and the anesthetist will "scrub up." You will lie on your side, or sit up, and the most you will feel is a small shot of local anesthetic in the skin and some pressure from the larger needle when the epidural space is entered. A fine catheter is then fed through the needle, the needle is removed, and the catheter, left in position, is strapped in place on your back and fixed on your shoulder. You will be given a test dose of the anesthetic; then the required amount will be injected through the catheter. The catheter stays in place throughout labor and delivery to allow a "topping up" of the initial dose to be given if necessary. The catheter is usually removed when you leave the delivery room.

Are there any risks involved with an epidural?

Sometimes complete pain relief is not achieved because of a technical problem, though this is very rare. What tends to happen is that a woman finds that about 1 square inch of flesh, often in one side of the groin, is sensitive and she still feels the pain there. It is tiresome if this occurs, but in 95 percent of women epidural anesthesia works completely.

About 5 percent of women undergoing epidurals experience a fall in blood pressure as mentioned above. But the technique has now been refined so that this no longer represents a problem.

Another complication associated with epidurals is that for some hours after birth, a percentage of women have a headache. It can be relieved by lying flat, or it may require medication.

Epidural anesthesia will *not* lead to infection, paralysis of the legs, or loss of bladder or bowel control after delivery.

OTHER FORMS OF ANESTHESIA

Spinal anesthesia

Spinal anesthesia is seldom used today, as it requires that the spinal fluid itself be entered. It is only given as a single shot (no "topping up"), which lasts for about 2 hours. It works very rapidly and may be useful in an emergency situation when there is not sufficient time for an epidural. Although spinal anesthesia is effective, it is more difficult to control and there is some risk of infection.

General anesthesia

General anesthetics are still administered in obstetrics for caesarean-section surgery, or for instrumental deliveries where, for example, the mother has severe hypertension or if forceps delivery has been attempted but the obstetrician has to turn to an emergency caesarean. A general anesthetic for a pregnant woman in labor must always be given by a skilled anesthetist as it can be hazardous. When pregnant, your stomach empties very slowly and there is always a danger of your inhaling vomit while you are unconscious. The anesthetist will constantly check for such a situation. General anesthetic agents present the additional hazard of crossing the placenta and temporarily sedating the baby.

Caudal anesthesia

For this procedure, an anesthetic agent is injected into the epidural space but the approach is different. The needle is passed through the lower spine via the gluteal cleft (up through the buttocks). However, the technique is seldom used because there is a greater risk of infection in this area.

Pudendal block

This form of anesthesia is used with an instrumental or forceps delivery, if you have not been given an epidural. The pudendal nerve controls pain at the outlet of the vagina, vulva, and pelvic floor, where the forceps are used. A needle is put in, with a special guard, through the vagina (or through the buttocks) and a local anesthetic is given at the level of the pudendal nerve. This ensures a painless forceps delivery, though it does not dull the pain of the contractions.

Local anesthesia

No episiotomy should ever be done without perineal infiltration. This is a painless injection in the perineal area (between the vagina and the anus). The local anesthetic will not harm the baby, as delivery is imminent, and there is little time for the pain-killing agents to enter the bloodstream and cross the placenta.

DELIVERY

The second stage of labor is involved with the delivery of the baby. It covers the time between reaching full dilation of the cervix (10 centimeters) and the expulsion of the baby. The doctor, nurse, and the mother herself can usually tell when the second stage is beginning, as the nature of the contractions changes. You will begin to experience the urge to bear down because of the pressure of the baby's head on your rectum. You feel a change in your breathing. You want to push. If the membranes have remained unruptured, they usually will break now.

On inspection of your vaginal area, it will be found that crowning has occurred. Your anus may extend widely. You will be taken to the delivery room (or you will stay in the birthing room but the bed will be prepared for delivery). Most women are still delivered on their backs, with their legs elevated in stirrups attached to the delivery bed. In birthing beds, you are allowed to deliver sitting upright, which is a position preferred by some women.

Tribal women in Africa deliver in the squatting position and there is a lot to be said for having gravity on your side. Why, you wonder, do we continue to keep women on their backs with their legs elevated? For the obstetrician there are many advantages to delivering a woman this way. If we have to use any instruments, it means there is no need for hasty changes of position. If yours is a very large baby, there is the possible hazard of the baby's shoulders becoming stuck during delivery. The legs-elevated position gives your doctor or midwife a good vantage of the perineum at all times. It enables us to move as we need to in order to turn the baby's head down to face the floor once the head has been delivered, so the shoulders can emerge.

In a normal delivery, the baby's head appears first. Once the head has been delivered, your doctor or midwife will gently depress it toward the floor, which lets the shoulders be born. They may ask you to control your pushing at this stage, to prevent your tearing. Once the baby has been expelled, the umbilical cord will be clamped twice and cut between the clamps. The baby's mouth and nose will be gently suctioned of mucus. Then the baby will be given to you to hold or to rest on your abdomen. If you do not feel strong enough, the baby can be placed on a heated pediatric table. Most babies cry immediately at birth or very shortly thereafter. But if your doctor is suctioning out the mouth and nose of mucus, do not panic if you do not hear a cry right away.

Will you have an episiotomy?

Episiotomy is the incision made in the perineum, between the vagina and the anus, to prevent this area from tearing during delivery. It is *not* done routinely in most medical centers; however, it is quite common. Usually it is necessary with a first baby, but not so vital in a second or subsequent pregnancy when the perineum can be massaged away from the baby's head.

An episiotomy must be performed with a breech or forceps delivery, because of the extra room required. In subsequent pregnancies, a previous episiotomy will not give you any problems. The scar cannot tear. Whether you have a repeat episiotomy will depend solely on the conduct of your current pregnancy.

At a certain point in delivery, the perineum is extended by the advancing baby's head. The episiotomy is done at this time. You will be given a local anesthetic prior to the procedure. The skin is incised at midline or off to one side. You will not feel any pain and, after the delivery of the baby and the placenta, your doctor will repair the incision, which takes about 5 minutes. We use absorbable gut for the stitches, so you will not have to have the stitches taken out.

The procedure is valuable not only because it prevents tearing, but because it takes pressure off the baby's head. It will also help prevent problems of vaginal collapse in older age, and it will mean you have a firm vagina after the birth.

Breech delivery

A breech delivery means that the lower part of the baby (buttocks) comes out first. As I explained earlier, only 2 to 3 percent of babies are in breech position at the end of pregnancy, as they will have been turned late in the third trimester either on their own or by external cephalic version (see page 212). If your baby has remained in a breech position, whether you will be able to have a natural delivery or should have a caesarean section will depend on your obstetrician's viewpoint, and on various medical factors concerning your pregnancy. The pendulum swings back and forth over which method is best for a breech birth. These days, we seem to be back to allowing natural deliveries. But this is still controversial. If the baby is not over 8 pounds or under 5½ pounds, then it may be safely delivered vaginally—provided, too, that the baby's neck is not hyperextended (the head is tipped back). If your doctor suspects hyperextension after feeling your abdomen, it can be confirmed by X ray before or during labor.

As I have previously said, the main thrust of obstetrics today is toward assuring the safety and health of your baby. The method of delivery will not, therefore, depend solely on the procedure preferred by either you or your doctor.

For vaginal delivery, labor in a breech birth will be identical to normal labor. The delivery itself should also be normal, except that once the trunk, arms, and legs are delivered, your doctor will probably use forceps to help deliver the baby's head. You will need an episiotomy for this procedure.

Why do we have to use forceps in a breech birth? The baby's head has to be delivered *very* slowly and forceps are used to help your doctor achieve sufficient control and to prevent sudden decompression should the head suddenly pop out. Forceps, as you will see below (page 272) are not used to pull the baby out, but to protect its head from injury.

What if your doctor does not use forceps for a breech delivery? Some doctors prefer not to use forceps and they can achieve the same amount of control with their hands. The obstetrician places his or her hands on the baby's head in a certain way, known as a Mauriceau-Smellie-Veit maneuver: The fingers of one of the doctor's hands go in the baby's mouth and onto its cheekbones, the other hand goes over the baby's shoulders, and the head is then delivered in a controlled manner (as effective as a forceps delivery). The decision for the best and safest route will be made by your doctor, who will discuss his or her methods with you at the time. There is a tendency to deliver first-pregnancy breech births by caesarean section, as the pelvis is untried.

Because of the potential problems with a breech vaginal delivery, it is always worth having a pediatrician present so any complications in the birth can be remedied as quickly as possible.

Multiple deliveries

The management of a twin delivery is approached as if there were two single babies to deal with. So, if one is a normal vaginal delivery, it does not follow that the other one will be. However, the commonest way for twin babies to present for birth is for both to be head down. Then delivery is about the same as for a normal pregnancy. The second twin usually comes 8 to 10 minutes after the first, but time is not important as long as the second baby's heart rate remains normal.

Once the first baby is delivered, if the second baby is not head down (but oblique or transverse), then your doctor can correct its position either by external cephalic version, through the abdomen, or by turning the baby with an internal version. The second pregnancy's membranes are ruptured and the doctor finds one of the baby's feet and turns it manually into the correct position. Twin deliveries have recently become safer since the exact position of the second baby and its condition can be confirmed by ultrasound machines and fetal monitors used on the labor floor.

If there should be three or more babies, it is more likely that you will have a caesarean section, to ensure their safe delivery, though some doctors will deliver triplets vaginally.

The hospital, too, must be adequately prepared for multiple deliveries because there is a chance that the babies will be small and more than one incubator will be required. When the South African sextuplets were born, I was working at the hospital at the time and their obstetrician was a colleague of mine. Needless to say it was a dramatic time, made more so by the fact they needed six teams of pediatricians and nurses, six incubators, and six resuscitators!

FORCEPS DELIVERY

Is there any risk in a forceps delivery?

Some women feel a sense of failure if they have a forceps delivery, as if it implied they were unable to push out the baby. Or they may imagine that forceps were used only because the doctor was in a hurry to get the delivery over with. Neither of these contentions is valid. Since so much undue worry can be attached to the idea of a forceps delivery, I want to set the picture straight here.

Forceps, or instrumental, deliveries have been practiced since the sixteenth century. There are many different types of forceps available. These metal blades are very simple in design and work very efficiently. One of their advantages is that they form a protective metal shield around the baby's head and, if there is any pulling, the forceps puts the pressure on the solid bone at the base of the head, rather than on the soft cranial bones at the top of the skull, thus *preventing* brain damage. In fact, forceps are mostly used in very high-risk pregnancies, or where the baby is immature, so as *not* to permit damage to the baby's brain.

Some of the bad press about forceps came about over a procedure used in the past, called "high forceps delivery," which is no longer practiced. In this case, the baby's head had not engaged in the pelvis and the forceps had to go high into the vagina to reach the head. A lot of trauma could be caused to the mother's tissue and to the baby as well. Today, forceps are only used if the baby's head is already engaged and at a low level in the pelvis.

What are the indications for the use of forceps?

Forceps are used only with proper medical indications in the second stage of labor when the cervix is fully dilated. One of these indications is fetal distress in the second stage. If the baby is in the breech position, forceps will be used on the after-coming head. If the baby is very immature, then forceps will be needed to protect its head. If the baby's head is in an unsuitable position for natural delivery, then forceps can be used to rotate the head to a suitable position.

There are also maternal reasons for using forceps: these include illnesses such as heart disease or hypertension, or severe maternal distress—conditions that require a shortened second stage of labor. Forceps can help lessen both the amount of time the second stage will take and the amount of effort exerted by the mother. Still another reason for the use of forceps is that a small percentage of women who have had epidural anesthesia may require assistance in pushing the baby out.

Certain conditions have to be met before a forceps delivery can be made. For example, your cervix must be fully dilated (second stage); the baby's head must be deeply engaged; your bladder must be emptied (catheterized); you will need suitable analgesia (such as an epidural or a pudendal block); and you will also have to have an episiotomy.

What happens during a forceps delivery?

By the second stage of labor, you will be in the delivery room, your legs will be elevated, and you will have been prepared for delivery in the usual way. The episiotomy will be performed; the required form of pain relief will be administered. Then the obstetrician places one hand alongside the baby's head and inserts one of the metal blades along the palm of the hand until it covers the head. The hand is removed and the procedure repeated at the opposite side of the baby's head. The blades will remain open and without pressure until the obstetrician is confident that they are equally balanced. The doctor locks the blades in position and, with each of your contractions, he or she pulls on the blades so the baby's head moves down the vaginal canal. Once the head appears, the blades are opened and removed. Delivery takes place in the normal fashion.

One woman asked me recently why the obstetrician cannot do this maneuver with his or her hands and why blades must be used? Human hands cannot get high enough into the vagina to protect the baby's head (see page 272). In breech delivery the hand maneuver can be used, for your doctor will be able to make use of the baby's shoulders and trunk to control delivery. For forceps delivery of the head, the blades are longer, stronger, and can perform this function without traumatizing the baby. Any marks on the baby's face usually disappear within hours.

Caesarean section

Who will have a caesarean section?

Let me first explain that caesarean deliveries are only performed for certain very definite indications. Contrary to much contemporary criticism, *maternal age* is *not* one of them. These indications do include a contracted pelvis or a very large baby, placenta previa, abnormal fetal position such as a transverse lie, fetal distress in labor, cord prolapse (umbilicus drops into the vagina before or during labor), severe high blood pressure in the mother, and cases in which the mother has had two previous caesareans, or a previous caesarean by classical caesarean section (in the upper part of uterus). A number of midforceps deliveries are also being replaced by caesarean section.

There has been much controversy in the press and negative public opinion about the allegedly accelerating rate of caesarean sections performed in the U.S. today. This criticism might have once been valid, but the rate is now declining and the latest statistics for the U.S. show that from 1981 to 1982 the rate of caesareans stood at only 16 percent in the nation overall, although the total number has increased.

In obstetric science the 1970s, as I have mentioned, was the decade of the fetus. We turned our concern from the fate of the mother and directed our energies and resources into improving the condition and health of the fetus. The rise in indications for caesarean section has resulted largely from that shift in emphasis.

There are also sociological and ethical reasons. We all have smaller families these days, and no one is likely to feel content to simply give birth to a baby with no regard for its condition, mental abilities, and strength to survive the years. In the past, as most people are aware, mothers gave birth to many more babies because the life expectancy of those children was far lower. At present, we want quality babies, not quantity.

When you are looking at the statistics, do not forget that at least one-third of the caesareans you read about are *repeat* caesareans; one-third are being done because the baby is too big or the pelvis is too small, or the baby is in the wrong position; fetal distress accounts for about 10 percent of the total; and the rest are performed for reasons that are varied.

Once a caesarean always a caesarean?

A lot of patients have been told that once they have had a caesarean they must have all future babies in the same fashion. But I wish to emphasize that these days that statement is definitely *not true*. You might have to have a repeat caesarean, of course, if you previously had a classical caesarean section, in which the cut went through the top part of the uterus; if a T-incision was made (the incision began in the lower segment but was extended into the upper segment of the uterus); if the first caesarean was done because your pelvis was too small; or if the pregnancy you are in now exhibits another unavoidable indication such as placenta previa. Otherwise, you should be able to have a vaginal delivery like that of any other normal pregnancy.

Vaginal delivery after previous caesarean section

If your doctor refuses to consider vaginal delivery after a previous caesarean section, for no valid reason, you may have to change doctors—unless, of course, the idea of a second caesarean does not disturb you. Some women find that elective caesarean the second time around is a relatively painless procedure that is easy to recover from, and they do not find the surgical intervention unpleasant. This is particularly true of women who learn they can have caesarean by epidural anesthesia, which means they can be awake during the operation and will see the baby the minute it is born. Some women, who may have had a difficult and long first labor that ended in emergency caesarean anyway, are quite grateful to contemplate the thought of elective caesarean without those complications.

All women have different priorities and interests regarding birth. I would no more consider forcing a woman to have a vaginal delivery after a previous caesarean than I would consider forcing her to do the opposite.

If you are going to have vaginal delivery after a previous caesarean section, you will have to be delivered in a hospital capable of handling a prompt emergency caesarean if it becomes necessary. Having said that, do not be afraid—despite any horror stories you may have heard. There is no increased maternal mortality for women who have had previous caesareans, and fetal mortality is no higher than in other pregnancies.

Your doctor will first have to investigate whether you are a candidate for vaginal delivery. He or she will watch you very carefully in labor. You will be able to go into labor naturally, but after admission to the hospital, you will be treated like a *potential* caesarean patient. You must not eat or drink, your blood will be cross-matched, and you will not be allowed to have an epidural during labor, so that the pain of uterine scar rupture will not be masked. You will be monitored very carefully.

What about possible rupture of the uterine scar? Rupture is very uncommon, but as your pregnancy advances after the thirtieth week, your doctor will check your uterus for tenderness and will ask you about any pain or bleeding. If you had a previous *classical* caesarean section, there is a 5 percent chance that the scar will rupture, in which case you would have to have an elective repeat caesarean before labor begins—at about 38 or 39 weeks. If you had the standard lower-uterine caesarean section, the incidence of scar rupture is 1 percent and such rupture can only occur *during* labor. You must alert your doctor the minute you are in labor. In the first stage of labor, you will be checked for any excess vaginal bleeding and your pulse rate will be monitored closely for a sudden jump. You will only be allowed a short second stage to reduce the amount of strain on the scar. Forceps should be used for the delivery to shorten the second stage. After delivery, your doctor will check the uterine scar to ensure that it is intact by performing a vaginal examination.

How is a caesarean section performed?

A caesarean section means delivering a baby by abdominal surgery. It can be performed before or during labor. If it is done electively (not as an emergency) in a planned procedure, there must have been adequate testing beforehand to see that the fetal lungs are mature. This testing will be done by ultrasound and amniocentesis, near term (39 to 40 weeks).

The operation can be performed under a general anesthetic or with regional anesthesia, called an epidural (see pages 261–265). At Mount Sinai Hospital two thirds are now done under epidural anesthesia. Doctors prefer to use this form of anesthesia, if possible, because it does not cause depression in the baby and there is almost no risk to the mother. (The greatest risk to the mother in a caesarean operation is from the general anesthetic, because of the possible danger of inhalation of stomach contents.) Epidural anesthesia enables the mother to enjoy the experience of birth.

Many women wonder how they can be awake during an abdominal surgical procedure. You will not see the actual surgery, so do not worry. You lie on the operating table and your abdomen is cleansed. You may be given some oxygen to breathe through a mask. Then a screen will be placed to obscure your view of the lower part of your body and to keep the surgical area sterile. The incision is usually a "bikini cut" (in the area of the shaved pubic hair), so you will not have a disfiguring scar. It takes about 8 to 10 minutes from the time surgery commences to the moment when the baby is lifted out. It will then take about 30 minutes to sew you up. Altogether, a caesarean takes about an hour.

Not all hospitals allow husbands into the operating room during a caesarean, but some top medical schools now do so, provided the husbands have been to preparation classes.

How safe is a caesarean section?

In the last few years caesarean section has become a very safe procedure, and you have absolutely no need to fear it. I would, however, advise you to wait at least 6 months before you conceive again, so that the gap between operations (if you need a repeat one) is more than a year. Your uterus will heal rapidly, in about 3 to 4 months.

When will you be able to hold your baby?

There is an increasing awareness of the importance of bonding between the baby and its parents in those first few moments after delivery. At Mount Sinai Hospital we now allow husbands to be present at the delivery, even for a caesarean section. Immediately after either vaginal or caesarean delivery, the mother is given her baby so she can hold it on her stomach and put it to the breast if she wishes. Both parents can touch and caress the baby and hear its first cry. It is a very important intimate and indefinably special moment between husband and wife, between parents and baby.

After these first few minutes, the nurse places the baby on a warmer. The pediatrician will check the baby for its alertness and will apply eye drops or cream to prevent infection from gonorrhea. Such treatment is required by law, worldwide.

We have found that even when the baby is on the warmer the mother will find her baby's eyes; a form of eye-to-eye contact called an "eye dance." Increasingly obstetricians are joining in the belief, held by women for many years, that either heavy analgesia or denying the mother her desire to hold her baby from the very beginning may be detrimental to bonding. (However, should you have to have a caesarean section under a general anesthetic, or if your baby is rushed to the intensive care unit, you should not worry that bonding cannot be made up later.)

While the baby is with the pediatrician, your episiotomy will be sewn up. Then, before you are taken to the recovery room, the baby will be handed back to you and you can keep it in your arms or at the breast for about 20 minutes in the recovery room. By this time the baby has been identified and tagged. But the baby must go up to the nursery to be weighed, and both you and your husband will be eager to know the weight. Once you reach your hospital room the baby will be given back to you again. There will be plenty of quiet time in which to get acquainted. It may even be valuable to use that short time while the baby is in the nursery to reorient your mind and ponder the recent exciting events.

Most hospitals and medical centers now have "rooming-in"

privileges (which means you can keep the baby with you in your room most of the time). Today, up to 80 percent of women request rooming-in, and more and more hospitals are being equipped with single rooms where the mother can keep the baby at all times if she wishes. More hospitals are also allowing sibling visits. The children usually should be over 2 years of age. Sometimes a cot is even put in the room so that the husband can sleep over if he wants to.

STILLBIRTH

The death of an infant before it is born, known as *death in utero*, is tragic, but fortunately it is a rare occurrence and one that is declining with improvements in modern obstetrics. A stillbirth is defined as any baby that dies after 28 weeks of pregnancy and before the end of labor. (Before the twenty-eighth week, its death is termed a miscarriage.)

The incidence of stillbirth is decreasing for several reasons that have to do with our better understanding of fetal well-being and with improved parental education; though the foremost reason is probably the implementation of comprehensive prenatal care, together with the systems that have been devised to identify high-risk pregnancies.

Some of the other more common causes for stillbirth in the past are now being eradicated as general medicine improves. A maternal illness such as diabetes used to be a major cause but no longer has such a devastating effect on pregnancy. Congenital abnormalities that might have led to a stillbirth are now detected early by amniocentesis or ultrasound. (If an abnormality is discovered, the mother may opt for an induced abortion, or *in utero* surgery may be performed to correct the abnormality before birth.)

Rh disease used to be a common cause of death *in utero* but this is being eliminated by the administration of Rhogam to Rh-negative mothers after a pregnancy, abortion, or amniocentesis; or, if the mother is already sensitized, then intrauterine transfusion is now possible to save the baby's life (see page 121).

There is, however, one condition that is still unpredictable and that can lead to rapid unexpected death of an infant: separation of the placenta (abruptio placentae). Unfortunately its cause is not known, and its occurrence cannot be predicted. However, for some as yet unknown reason this cause of stillbirth is also becoming rarer. Knots or accidents to the umbilical cord can cause the death of an infant, though such accidents are very rare.

Can your baby become entangled in the cord and suffer strangulation? The pulsations of the blood circulating in the cord prevent it from drawing tightly around the baby's neck. So, if the cord has wrapped itself around the baby's neck once, it will not be strangled. If the cord is twice around the neck, then it can tighten during labor when pressure is applied to the cord. But this condition can be diagnosed in plenty of time to prevent problems, as it will show up as a certain pattern on the fetal monitor. We do not as yet have ultrasound machines refined enough to show the exact image of the cord either knotted or wrapped twice around the baby's neck. However, in the near future there will no doubt be a more refined machine that will show us such minute detail, as ultrasound technology is improving so rapidly.

When stillbirth does occur, it is generally caused by poor functioning of the placenta (placental insufficiency, or growth retardation). Babies so affected usually do not die suddenly, without any prior warning. If you are aware of the importance of fetal movements (see pages 227–231) you will no doubt alert your doctor if there is any noticeable decrease.

How is stillbirth diagnosed?

Usually the mother is the first person to suspect that something irreversible has happened to her baby when she notices an absence of fetal movements over a period of 12 to 24 hours. She may no longer feel pregnant, her breasts may be less swollen. If your baby has unfortunately died *in utero* it will not be dangerous to you, though your emotional response, sorrow, and sense of inadequacy, together with the psychological effect of knowing you are carrying a dead baby, will not make your treatment easy.

It used to be very difficult to confirm infant death *in utero*. Even though the doctor would not be able to hear the fetal heart through the stethoscope, that was not enough reason to pronounce the baby dead. We used to do a series of X rays to watch for bone changes in the fetus, but this took time to develop—as long as 3 to 6 weeks. Fortunately, we now have ultrasound, so these X rays are no longer required. Ultrasound is safe and can be repeated daily if necessary. Using an ultrasound machine, it can be seen immediately whether the baby's heart is beating, and whether there are any fetal movements.

Up to 10 years ago, if *in utero* death was diagnosed, you would then have had to wait for the onset of labor, which might have taken a few weeks. We could not induce labor with oxytocin, as that only worked on women who were naturally ready for labor. Your doctor would not have been able to break your water because of the risk of infection to you. We used to use all sorts of drugs to try to induce early labor. But, fortunately, we now have prostaglandins, which when placed in the vagina in sufficient quantity will cause cervical changes in any woman at any stage of pregnancy, and will induce labor. (I mentioned a similar use of prostaglandins in inducing early abortions on pages 19–20.) They are very effective and can be used safely, particularly in cases of stillbirth.

The induction of labor must be done in a hospital. Your blood will be checked beforehand for its coagulation profile, since in a very small percentage of women who suffer a stillbirth, a rare but potentially serious blood disorder known as a "coagulation defect" may develop. This occurs a couple of weeks after the death, and is caused by the absorption of fetal products into your circulation. It may result in bleeding into the skin, or from your nose or vagina.

After delivery and once pathology reports have come through, your doctor should take time to explain to you exactly why your baby died, so that you can approach your grief as pure bereavement, rather than overloading it with guilt or feelings of personal failure. Do not hesitate to see the baby or to find out its sex, if it will help you.

C H A P T E R

6

After Delivery

The time after delivery is known as the postpartum period, or the puerperium. It begins once the baby and the placenta have been delivered. Some books try to define a time limit, from 10 days to 4 or 6 weeks, but it is impossible to do so, as it depends on the time required for the body to revert to its prepregnant state, and this time varies tremendously among individual women. Traditionally, however, you see your doctor 6 weeks after birth for a final checkup, because your reproductive tract should be back to normal by then.

What changes are happening to your body?

Uterus: The uterus is quite a unique organ, as it has grown to weigh almost 2 pounds during pregnancy and will now shrink back to its prepregnant weight of about 4 ounces. It is the only organ in the body that can go through such changes. Immediately after delivery your abdomen will look flatter, as the uterus begins to shrink rapidly, contracting down to the level of the umbilicus. From the second day on, it shrinks at a rate of one-half inch a day. By the twelfth day you will no longer be able to feel the uterus in your abdomen. The nurses and doctor will be checking for the decrease in the height of your uterus when they feel your abdomen during the puerperium.

At this time there will also be a discharge of blood and uterine lining (decidua) from the uterus. This discharge, known as lochia, is perfectly normal and your doctor or nurse will be checking your sanitary pad at frequent intervals to make sure that it is present and that it does not have a foul odor (which could be a sign of infection).

The lochia remains quite red for the first 3 to 6 days after delivery because it contains blood from the big veins in the uterus that have been supplying the placenta.

After about a week, the lochia will still be present but paler in color, because the venous openings in the uterus are closing off as the uterus shrinks. The pale color is also due to the white blood cells that have rushed to the uterus to defend you against infection should it occur. The paler lochia flow may normally continue for up to 6 weeks or even longer.

There may be times when the flow increases after nearly disappearing. This will probably be due to extra exertion once you have returned home. After breast-feeding, the lochia may flow more freely, as stimulation of the breasts causes uterine contractions, which will squeeze out more blood. The lochia is a healthy sign, and not anything to fear.

When should you worry about the amount of lochia?

If the discharge becomes foul-smelling or begins to become red, heavy, and floods down your legs, then you should lie down and call your doctor. The bad odor may mean infection, which can be treated with certain safe antibiotics, even if you are breast-feeding. The flooding of blood may be a sign of postpartum hemorrhage, which can happen if part of the placenta has been retained. However, this is fortunately a rare occurrence, as part of your doctor's or midwife's duty is to check the afterbirth on delivery and see that it is complete. Postpartum hemorrhage is treated by D & C (dilation and curettage) to check for retained placenta. It will not affect a future pregnancy.

What changes are occurring in the vagina and cervix?

After delivery the vagina is lax and distended. It may have stretched up to 30 centimeters to enable the baby's head to pass through, and very likely you have had an episiotomy if this was your first baby. Within a few days the vagina recovers its tone, though it never regains the little corrugations that it had in the prepregnant state (this is not a significant change that will affect your life in the long run).

The cervix, which is loose and hanging at first, will be closed again in 6 or 7 days. So, within the first week after delivery you have to be particularly careful about hygiene to avoid infection, as the open cervix can be a tract for infection from the vagina into the uterine cavity. Infection is quite simply prevented by washing yourself down with a jet of water after any visit to the bathroom, always wiping your anus from the front to the back, and using sterile sanitary pads, not tampons, to absorb the lochia. You must also pay careful attention to the episiotomy sutures, and to cleansing the perineal area. Because of the risk of infection, intercourse is discouraged for the first 5 weeks after delivery. By the fifth week, your vagina should also be tight again and the episiotomy will be healed.

Will you have after-birth pains?

After-birth pains are uncommon after a first baby, but following a second or subsequent baby you may have contractions as painful as those at the height of labor, for some 48 to 72 hours after delivery. We are not certain why this happens, but it probably has to do with the uterus returning to normal. You may need Tylenol or stronger medication if the pains bother you seriously.

If you have had a caesarean section, you still get after-birth pains in a second or subsequent pregnancy and this can be aggravated by distension of the bowel. You can relieve the gas pains that usually occur on the second or third day by sucking peppermint, drinking peppermint tea, or taking a laxative or an antispasmodic. Your doctor may order an enema or the insertion of a flatus tube to get rid of the gas and decrease the bowel distension.

Within a day or so after vaginal or caesarean delivery you may find you are passing a lot of urine. The extra fluid that accumulated in the bloodstream and tissues during pregnancy is being excreted, and with it any swelling of the hands or feet should slowly disappear. Leg swelling, however, may take a full week to diminish.

The episiotomy scar

How long will the stitches hurt? If you had an epidural anesthetic for labor, or a local anesthetic for the episiotomy, you will find the sutures do pull once the analgesic effect has worn off. Within 24 to 48 hours, however, they should no longer be painful. You can take Tylenol to ease the discomfort, or a local anesthetic spray may be used on the sutures. The stitches will not have to be taken out, as they are absorbed by the body and fall away. If the stitches continue to pull, twice-daily sitz baths will help to relieve the tension, as will sitting on a round rubber air tube.

When can you have a bath?

Because it takes a week for the cervix to close, you will not want to take a bath and risk having the water rise through the cervix until at least this first week has passed. You may shower and wash your hair from the first day after a vaginal delivery. If you have had a caesarean section, you should not wet your sutures for 6 days, so you will not be able to take a full shower until a week has passed. You can wash the perineal area and any other part of the body, in a hand basin. You may also wash your hair if you can find a friend, husband, or nurse to help you bend over the basin.

Will you get the "blues"?

Sometimes, on the second or third day after delivery, mothers become weepy or depressed, which is a condition that is quite normal after birth and is generally known as the "blues." You may feel watery eyed, your lips may start to tremble as you talk to a friend or family member on the telephone, particularly if you have a younger child at home, and it will take very little to bring on floods of tears that appear to have no end. With some women, this condition may coincide with the newborn infant's becoming slightly jaundiced (yellow), which is a mild condition that happens to many newborns and is not something to worry about. But, when you are told on the third day that your baby has jaundice, you may be convinced something is seriously wrong that the doctors have been hiding from you. Feelings of self-pity, helplessness, and inadequacy in the face of too much to cope with can overwhelm you at this point.

There is little that can be done medically to help. You will require warm reassurance and sympathetic nursing; also, it is hoped that your husband will be supportive during this minor crisis. Do not ask for Valium (diazepam) or try to dampen the feelings. They will work their way through you and probably will not last more than 24 hours. Many adjustments are happening to your body. You are suffering the psychological separation of no longer having the baby inside the uterus, and although we are not yet certain of its exact cause, the "blues" probably have to do with changing brain metabolism, which, as I mentioned before, is thought to be responsible for the major mood changes in the different trimesters of pregnancy.

How soon can you exercise?

After a normal vaginal delivery you should try to get out of bed after a few hours, to improve your circulation and help prevent thrombosis. You can begin some gentle postnatal exercises such as those to build strength in the pelvic floor (see page 198) on the first day. You will no doubt want to do everything possible to help your vagina regain its natural tone and tightness, and to encourage the uterus to shrink in size. (Contrary to some popular opinion, it is not essential to lie on your stomach to encourage the uterus back into proper shape.)

Regular heavy exercises such as situps and straight-leg raises should not be begun for 3 weeks, as your stomach muscles will be very stretched after the pregnancy, and you will be tired. Although you want to restore muscle tone, it is not a good idea to overstretch your muscles until they have had time to adjust. If you have had an up-and-down caesarean section, you should not start regular exercises for 6 weeks. But, if yours was a bikini incision, you may also begin exercises after 3 weeks.

Rest and visitors

It is very pleasant to have visitors, to show off the baby, and discuss the details of the birth. It may be better, however, not to have too many visitors but rather to use this special time well, to rest, to bond quietly and slowly with your baby.

Should your baby be circumcised?

There is a fair amount of controversy over circumcision at the moment, so I would advise you to discuss it with your husband and doctor before the birth in case you have a boy. They will want to know in the hospital very shortly after delivery whether the procedure is to be done, and you may be in no mood to make such a decision then.

Unless circumcision is part of a religious ceremony, the procedure is usually done by the obstetrician (not the pediatrician) on the second or third day after delivery, providing the baby's pediatrician agrees. It is done without an anesthetic, but the baby must not be fed beforehand or it could lead to vomitus being inhaled. It is not traumatic for your baby to be circumcised. The procedure takes in all about 3 to 4 minutes, and it will not delay your leaving the hospital even on the same day. The nurse will check for any bleeding and will instruct you how to care for the wound when you change the diapers. It only requires Vaseline gauze on the penis at each diaper change for 3 to 4 days.

Will you lose your hair after the birth of your baby?

Some women may have thinning of the hair in the few weeks after delivery. It is not uncommon for some to come out as you brush or comb your hair, and, though this can be understandably disturbing, it does not mean you are going bald. We do not know the exact cause of the hair fall, but it is unusual for it to become a major problem and it ordinarily stops within a few months (or when you finish breast-feeding).

Why do puerperal fevers develop and how dangerous are they?

A slight fever after the delivery can lead to misery and disappointment if you are not permitted to breast-feed your baby. Babies are thought to be immune from our infections for the first 6 months of their life, but as a precautionary measure most hospitals will not allow the mother to breast-feed if she is running a fever (and sometimes she may not even be permitted to hold the baby). If this situation does arise for you, it can be minimized by sympathetic nursing care and you should be encouraged and helped to express your milk, either manually or with an electric breast pump, every 4 hours, so that once the fever passes you will be able to put the baby straight back to the breast without a problem.

Some women develop a mild fever due to the stress of labor. It appears soon after delivery and will last for about 12 hours. Other women may come into labor with a fever from a cold or flu, and the postpartum fever will then be a continuation from the prior infection.

A common fever occurs 2 or 3 days after delivery. It used to be known as "milk fever," since it came at the same time as the milk was filling the breasts, leaving them hard and engorged. If your breasts are very tender and hard, then the cause of your slight fever is probably not difficult to trace. It can be relieved by emptying the breasts yourself.

Another early developing fever is "puerperal fever" itself, which is the once dread disease that caused the deaths of so many women after childbirth in previous centuries. Puerperal fever is caused by an infection in the uterus. Presumably bacteria from around the anus or perineum enter the uterus through the open cervix. It presents at first with a low temperature and your lochia may be offensive in odor, heavier, and brighter red in color. Your doctor will take a culture through the cervix from the uterus, using a sterile speculum. (The culture must not be taken from the vagina, where bacteria are always present.) The culture will be sent for bacteriological analysis and, if positive, you will be treated with antibiotics that are safe even if you want to continue breast-feeding.

From the third to the fifth day after delivery, if your bladder has been catheterized during labor, you might develop a bladder infection known as cystitis. The infection may be accompanied by a fever, shaking, and chills, and you will pass urine more often than usual. You may associate the word *cystitis* with a burning sensation from passing urine, yet it is quite common, after childbirth, to suffer the infection *without* this frequent symptom. The trauma of delivery seems to remove the sensation of discomfort from the bladder. If cystitis is suspected, you will probably be asked to collect a clean midstream sample of your urine, which will be sent to the lab for a culture. Treatment is with antibiotics that are safe for use even if you intend to continue breast-feeding. Two or three weeks later you must have a follow-up urine culture to ensure that the infection has been eradicated.

The infection of either the episiotomy or caesarean-section wound can also lead to a fever. The pain will be regional and your doctor can diagnose it by checking for pus around the sutures. The treatment for infection of an episiotomy is twice-daily sitz baths with salt in the water. You will not be resutured and there is little to worry about, as the scar will heal itself in time. If the caesarean-section scar has become infected (usually around the fifth day after delivery), the wound will be inflamed, bright red, and there may be a collection of fluid under the stitches. Your doctor can lift a few stitches to allow the pus to come out. You will not need antibiotics and the procedure itself is not painful.

Venous thrombosis is one serious complication that can occur on the seventh or eighth day after delivery. Venous thrombosis is not the mild superficial redness of veins in your legs that is called phlebitis. (Phlebitis is not dangerous and can usually be treated simply by wearing support hose.) But this condition is a deep vein thrombosis that can appear any time after the fifth day, especially if you had surgery. It will be accompanied by a fever, you may notice a pain in the calf of one leg, and you may be tested by being asked to flex your leg to see if that causes the pain to recur.

If thrombosis is diagnosed, it must be vigorously treated with injections of heparin. You will have to remain in bed with your legs elevated, bandaged to the groin. The thrombosis might have occurred because of changes in blood coagulation associated with pregnancy. It is very serious if not treated immediately, for a piece of a clot from your leg can break off and flow through the bloodstream to the lungs, leading to chest pains and at worst coughing up of blood due to pulmonary embolism.

Fortunately the risk of such a condition is minimized now by adequate hydration (fluids) during labor and early ambulation from your bed after delivery. With a caesarean section, you are encouraged to walk around the bed on the first or second day after surgery and to practice deep breathing. For natural delivery, you should be out of bed after a few hours.

If you are being given heparin injections for this condition, you may continue to breast-feed your baby. But, once you are on the oral medication to anticoagulate the blood (Coumadin), you will have to discontinue breast-feeding since oral medication passes through into your milk.

One final cause of fever that may also occur late in the week after delivery, around the eighth day, is a breast abscess. Not the same as milk fever, this condition is caused by an infection in only one breast. You will have a localized bright red area, tender to the touch. If it is noticed early, before the accumulation of pus, treatment will be a high dose of penicillin by mouth. You must take the baby off the breast with the abscess, express the milk in that breast either manually or with an electric breast pump, and not put the baby back to that breast until the abscess is cleared up. If there is a delay in diagnosing the abscess, the accumulation of fluid in it may require surgical drainage, which has to be done under a general anesthetic. It is an unfortunate condition, but not unusual, and it does illustrate why you have to be meticulous about hygiene when you are breast-feeding, always washing the nipple and your hands before putting the baby's mouth to the breast.

What problems might you have with breast-feeding?

One of the functions of a good obstetrician or midwife is to help you with breast-feeding. There are many books and publications that emphasize the advantages of breast-feeding and you should perhaps read some of them before labor. It is well known, for example, that mother's milk is perfect for the baby in composition, temperature, and convenience.

There are very few women for whom breast-feeding is medically contraindicated, except those on drug therapy that cannot be stopped. If your baby has to spend considerable time in intensive care, you may not manage to keep up the milk supply in the first few days after the birth. If this happens, then the formulas available today to feed your baby will keep the baby in good health, and your child will not be disadvantaged later in life.

Your early milk contains substances needed for the baby's protection, from antibodies, to laxatives, to your own bacteria, which help guard it against infection in those early weeks. If you are ambivalent about breast-feeding, you can always nurse for only the first two or three weeks, and then take the baby off the breast. There is no evidence as yet regarding the optimal length of time to breast-feed. Much research is now being conducted into the composition of breast milk, and with the passage of time, I believe we will know more about the relative benefits of early and later breast-feeding. We do know that it has been shown to be beneficial in the prevention of breast cancer in your later years.

If you have any doubts or are feeling nervous about breast-feeding, you should contact the excellent La Leche League, either through their local branch listed in your telephone directory, or at their headquarters address: La Leche League International, 9616 Minneapolis Avenue, Franklin Park, IL 60131. They have leaflets and information on breast-feeding and can also put you in touch with local groups that will offer training and support for the nursing mother.

Often anxiety first sets in when you have gotten back home from the hospital and find yourself on your own with the baby. Suddenly what appeared to be an angel in the hospital turns into a monster. The baby cries through the night. Either you or your husband, or both, fear your milk supply is inadequate, which is why the baby is crying so much. That fear makes you decide to give up breast-feeding for the relative safety of the bottle, where you can see how much the baby has drunk and convince yourself or your husband that at least you are not starving the baby. Those first few days or weeks back home can be a very trying time, owing to lack of sleep and a totally disturbed domestic routine. If you have had any fears of being inadequate as a mother, they will come to the surface now. If your husband, for example, is convinced the baby cries because *you* cannot give it enough milk, how are you to argue the opposite? It can be difficult to rely on one's body in a way you have never had to depend upon it before. However, a phone call to a La Leche League representative in a moment of crisis may well soothe those worries and give you sufficient confidence to get through this difficult stage.

If you decide you cannot or do not wish to breast-feed, in most cases you will only need to wear a firm bra, and cut down on the amount of liquid you drink, for the milk to disappear or not start to flow. The effect of a firm bra is to suppress the milk lobules and prevent the establishment of lactation. However, if lactation has already begun, you may need some treatment to stop the flow of milk. Bromocryptine mesylate (Parlodel) will inhibit the secretion of prolactin, one of the main hormones responsible for lactation. Unlike estrogen, which used to be prescribed, the administration of bromocryptine mesylate has so far shown no long-term or harmful side effects.

When should you first put the baby to the breast?

Although there is no real secretion of milk for the first 3 days after birth, the baby will profit from being put to the breast after delivery, as the breasts contain colostrum. Colostrum has actually been in the breasts from midpregnancy. Putting the baby to the breast will encourage bonding between the two of you and help establish the baby's sucking motion.

The supply of breast milk responds to the baby's demands. The more the baby sucks, the more you produce. This supply-and-demand feature goes into action from the very beginning. When you gave birth, the estrogen in your blood decreased, which allowed the hormone prolactin to operate. Once the pro-lactin is active it causes milk to accumulate in the breasts, and once the baby sucks, oxytocin is released from the brain and helps to release the milk. As the baby sucks the length of the nipple into its mouth, the muscles around the milk lobules in the breasts are stimulated to squeeze out the milk (this is the "let-down" response). The same sucking action also helps your uterus to contract—which means your stomach will become flatter in a much shorter time.

During the first 3 days, the baby should be at the breast at least two or three times a day. Do not allow more than 10 minutes per breast each time. The nurses will help you place the nipple in the baby's mouth, but you will soon see that the baby clamps on like a magnet once shown the way. Do not get despondent if on the third day a setback seems to occur. This is the time that babies can develop jaundice; you may also be suffering the "blues," and end up feeling you just cannot cope with breast-feeding. The blues and the jaundice will pass. Do not let these immediate emotions affect what could be a long and wonderful relationship for you as a breast-feeding mother with her baby. It will all turn out right in the end. That there are no absolute rules is made obvious by conflicting advice from professionals. Once your lactation has been established, feeding should be on demand, or whenever the baby cries for these first few days, to help establish your bonding and ease its path into the world. When you are back home, you can try to adopt a routine that is more convenient to your life style, or you can continue to breast-feed on demand, as you wish.

If you develop cracked nipples, which can be quite painful, it will be from the direct effect of the baby's gums chewing on your nipples. This condition can usually be relieved by taking the baby off the breast in question for 24 hours. If *both* nipples are similarly affected, you may have to stop breast-feeding for 24 hours and express your breasts to stop them from getting too engorged and hard.

Will your breasts return to normal after breast-feeding?

Although your breasts were enlarged and heavier during pregnancy, and will probably be much larger now that you are breast-feeding, that is no guarantee that they will remain larger when you finish breast-feeding. There will usually be some permanent change in their size or shape, but quite what kind of change is unpredictable. Some women complain that they lost a once healthy bust after breast-feeding to become quite flat-chested; other women find their breasts increase in size after the baby is weaned. Remember that the breasts should be adequately supported during the heavier times so that the breast ligaments do not become overstretched.

Drugs and their effect on breast-feeding

Any drug you take into your body will be excreted in breast milk. Just as it was very important not to take medical or social drugs in early pregnancy, so it is equally important not to when breast-feeding. Over-the-counter medications such as antihistamine-containing cold cures, laxatives, and antacids, as well as sedatives, alcohol, cigarettes, marijuana, and diazepam (Valium) are all contraindicated.

I could give you an even longer list of drugs that cross to your milk, but you really do not need to know the names of each one, since all drugs cross.

What if you develop herpes after the birth?

If you get a herpes ulcer on your genitalia or lips, you will be isolated from other mothers in the hospital, but your baby will remain with you so that it does not come into contact with the other babies in the nursery. You may still breast-feed your baby, but you must pay strict attention to hand washing, and if you have oral herpes, you should wear a mask on your face so that the infant does not contract the virus. If you had herpes when you gave birth, you would have been delivered by cae-sarean section, and you may breast-feed.

If visitors or relatives have herpes, they should not visit you and the baby, nor should they even come into the hospital.

When can you go home?

After a vaginal delivery you will usually be allowed to go home on the third day. After a caesarean section, your stay will probably last for 5 days, depending on your recovery from surgery. Although there is a tendency in birthing clinics and some hospitals these days to send you home on the first day after a simple normal delivery, I advise you to wait the prescribed 3 days mainly because you need rest, and caring for a baby is much harder at home than in the hospital.

Moreover, various conditions that might need the attention of the hospital pediatrician tend to occur between 24 hours and the third day after delivery. This is particularly true of infant jaundice. With mothers going home earlier, we are now seeing babies being readmitted for bad cases of jaundice after several days at home. The delay in medical attention might lead to complications, or more problems with the quite common newborn jaundice than if it had been noticed and treated in the first few days of your baby's life. Also, if your baby has to be readmitted to the hospital once you have left the maternity ward, you will have to take the baby to a general pediatric ward where you will not be allowed to stay overnight.

Certain congenital disorders, such as a congenital hip defect or heart murmur, might also not be apparent in the baby until 24 to 48 hours have elapsed. If you take the baby home on the first day, such a defect might not be picked up for many weeks and this can have devastating effects. If hip dislocation is noticed within the first 24 hours after the baby's delivery, it can be corrected just by double-diapering. If there is a delay of several weeks before the pediatrician notices the condition, then surgery becomes a more likely corrective measure.

When can you have intercourse again?

Intercourse is discouraged for 5 weeks after delivery to deter infection and to allow time for the vagina to heal and regain its tone. It is actually a good idea to have intercourse, if possible, at about the fifth week, so that when you see your doctor for the final 6-week checkup you can report any problem (such as the episiotomy's being too tight), if one is discovered. You do not need contraception between the fifth and sixth week after delivery.

If you had an episiotomy, you might be nervous that sex will be painful. My advice is that if on commencing intercourse you feel very tight, suggest to your husband that he use a lubricant such as K-Y jelly and that he begin entering you very slowly and gently. Even if he cannot attain full penetration the first time, it does not mean you are irreparably or permanently affected. If you both take your return to lovemaking slowly, you should resume normal practice quite easily. However, if after a few efforts there is still a problem, you will be able to discuss this with your obstetrician at the final checkup.

You may find your libido rather low in the first few weeks after having the baby. This is partly due to the metabolic changes taking place in your brain as your body reverts to its prepregnant state, and partly due to the emotional overload you will be experiencing as you accustom yourself to life with the new baby. By the fifth or sixth week, your libido should have returned to normal. If it remains low for a longer period, there is nothing to worry about. You may be experiencing a particularly difficult period of readjustment to the new family, and to its psychological and emotional demands. However, if you feel serious problems are developing between your husband and yourself in this postpartum period, it might be advisable to seek out either marriage therapy or a group of similar new parents who are meeting to discuss and compare notes about this milestone event. Ask your doctor, local family therapist, women's group, or hospital for the name of such a group. You do not have to feel yours is the only marriage suffering from the strains of "bringing home baby"!

May you climb stairs after a caesarean section?

Some books imply that you should treat yourself as an invalid for the first few weeks after a caesarean section, and forbid climbing stairs or lifting. But I do not believe you should approach your recuperation this way. The biggest difference between you and the mother who had a vaginal delivery is that you had to stay in the hospital those extra days.

Like any new mother, you may be very tired when you first get home, particularly if the baby is up in the night. You will have to adjust to the lack of sleep. In your case, it will be aggravated by the fact that you are feeling weak after surgery. Be careful to eat well, rest in the daytime, and spend a couple of hours a day reading or doing whatever else you find relaxing.

I also suggest that you try to get out of the house, unless it is too cold, for a short walk each day so you'll begin to feel normal again as soon as possible. You may want to have someone in your house to help you.

If you have had a vertical caesarean skin incision, then you should not lift anything heavy for a month. But if you have had a bikini cut, you really do not need to treat yourself any differently from any other new mother. You may climb stairs, or lift your two-year-old if need be. The only limiting factor will be your own pain and tolerance for discomfort.

Can you go on a diet once the baby is born?

If you gained an average 25 to 30 pounds during your pregnancy, you should lose 16 pounds (7.5 kilograms) or more immediately after delivery (with the loss of amniotic fluid, extra blood, the baby itself, and the weight of the enlarged uterus). With exercise and careful control of what you eat, there is no reason your figure should not return to normal in a fairly rapid time.

If you are breast-feeding, a crash diet is not permitted, as a reliance on certain foodstuffs will affect the composition of your milk and thus your baby's health and condition. You must eat healthily and well while breast-feeding, as you did during pregnancy—with extra protein, milk, vegetables, and fresh fruit in your daily diet. Diet pills are most definitely not allowed, as they contain drugs that will be dangerous to your baby's health. You should, however, continue to take your prenatal vitamins.

When you stop breast-feeding you will lose a further 5 to 6 pounds. However, as the effect of breast-feeding is to use up many extra calories per day, providing food for both baby and you, you may find your waistline beginning to spread if you continue to eat the same diet after your baby is weaned. Once you have finally taken the baby off the breast, and you are fully recovered from the birth and the adjustment of your new life with the baby, then is the time to diet, following whatever sound dietary advice you wish.

Will your stretch marks disappear?

Marks on the breasts, thighs, and abdomen will become paler and may almost disappear, but they are likely to remain faintly visible for the rest of your life. Pigmentation of the nipples and of your abdomen below the umbilicus, may also remain a darker color. Certain body changes of pregnancy are permanent, but they tend to be quite insignificant.

Varicose veins usually disappear and should not be assessed for treatment until 6 months have passed after delivery. In all probability, they will have returned to normal by then. The same applies to hemorrhoids, which are really varicose veins of the anus.

When will your periods return?

The time that your periods return will depend most on whether you breast-feed or not. If you decide *not* to breast-feed, they usually return 8 to 10 weeks after delivery. Just as at other major times in your life, such as the beginning of menstruation, after an abortion, or with menopause, their pattern may be erratic—either much heavier, much lighter, or more or less painful. This does not mean they will be altered permanently.

Even when your menstruation does return you will not know for certain whether you are ovulating or not, especially if you are still breast-feeding. If you are breast-feeding, it may be some 14 to 16 weeks after delivery before the periods return, or they may not reappear until you wean the baby from the breast. That can mean you have no periods for as much as a year, or they may begin to come back as you slowly take the baby off the breast—for example, if you only give the baby a night and morning breast-feed.

The chances of becoming pregnant again within the first 4 months after delivery are very low, even if you are not breast-feeding, because ovulation is not likely to have started up again. However, as it is never certain whether you are ovulating or not, contraception should be used after your 6-week checkup, even if you are breast-feeding. There are still women who have babies spaced 9 to 12 months apart—who had no idea they had become pregnant again when they were breast-feeding.

What contraceptive method should you use?

You should discuss your future contraceptive method at the 6-week checkup with your obstetrician. If you are breast-feeding, oral contraceptives (the Pill) are not permitted, as the hormones will pass through to your milk and will suppress its production. Most women choose to be fitted with an IUD (intrauterine device) or a diaphragm. You will probably need a different-size diaphragm from the one you used before the pregnancy. Many women go up in size by 5 millimeters after birth. If you are not breast-feeding, you may start the Pill, and your first period will come at the end of your first packet.

Why do you need the doctor's final checkup?

Your last visit to your obstetrician for this birth will be at 6 weeks after delivery. If you have had a caesarean section, your scar will have been checked earlier, 2 weeks after leaving the hospital.

The doctor or nurse will now weigh you and check your blood pressure, which should be back to normal if it was raised because of your pregnancy. Your breasts will be examined for lumps (though this is not always done if you are breast-feeding, since lumps are not easy to interpret among the milk glands). You will have a pelvic examination to ensure that your episiotomy has healed well, that the vaginal inlet is adequate, that the cervix is closed, the uterus back to normal, and that the ovaries are normal. Sometimes a Pap smear is done because you will be due for one after the passage of the 9 months. Your future method of contraception will be discussed. And your doctor will no doubt discuss with you how you and your husband are adjusting to the new life with the baby, and how you are coping with breast-feeding. You may wish to bring up some of your worries, concerns, or just gratitude for the new life and discuss it with this partner, friend, and medical supporter with whom you have worked over 9 or more months to produce your wonderful, healthy, normal, and vital baby. It is a happy moment for both doctor and new mother.

The next chapters, of course, are out of my hands; they are yours alone. Learning to love your baby at home, as a member of your family, will be an exciting time for you. This is what makes my work as an obstetrician all the more rewarding; knowing the pleasure and satisfaction my work helps bring to the couples I meet in the course of a working life. And remember, by the time you are considering consulting your obstetrician about another baby, there will be yet more knowledge and even more refined techniques for understanding exactly what is happening during the long nine months of fetal life.

Index

weight loss after stopping, 301
Breast milk, 294, 295, 296
Breasts, 123
  abscess of, 293
  after breast feeding, 397
  changes in, 86
  examination of, 303-304
Breathing, 87, 205
Breech delivery, 268, 269-270
Breech position, 211
Bromocryptine mesylate, 295

Caesarean section, 274-278
  and breech births, 270
  care after, 289, 300-301
  and electronic fetal heart monitors, 253
  infection from, 292
  for multiple delivery, 271
  and placenta previa, 192, 209
Caffeine, 11, 122, 128, 138, 174, 194
Calcium, 126
Calisthenics, 197
Cancer, 5, 7, 44
Canker sore, 136
Car, see Automobile
Carrier screening, 76, 77
Castor oil, 133
Cat feces, 63
Cathode ray tube (CRT) terminals, 59
Caudal anesthesia, 266
Cell division, 69
Cephalic version, external, 269
Cephalosporins, 30
Cervix, 13, 286
  incompetent, 159-160
  opening during pregnancy, 21-22
Chickenpox, 132
Childbirth, see Delivery
Chlamydia, 25, 117
Cholasma, 86
Chloroquine, 151

Cholasma, 86
Cholera vaccine, 151
Chorionic membrane, 88
Chromosomal abnormality, 23, 27, 164
Chromosomal disorders, 78
  and miscarriages, 23, 26-27, 78
  see also Down's syndrome
Chromosomes
  analysis, 70-71, 84
  and autosomes, 68, 69, 73
  sex, 68, 69, 73
Cigarette smoking, 4, 7, 11, 34-35
Circumcision, 289-290
Cleft lip, 73
Cleft palate, 31, 73, 170
Clomid, 14, 164, 213
Clomiphene, 213
Clubfoot, 73, 170
Coal-tar-based dyes, 65
Cocaine, 37, 39
Coffee, 122, 138
Colace, 132
Cold remedies, 4, 31
Colds, 131
Cold sore, 136
Colostrum, 155, 205, 296
Communicable diseases, 4
Conception, 8
  difficulties, and marijuana, 7, 36
  and exercise, 53-54
Condoms, 12
Condyloma acuminatum, 50
Congenital heart disease, 170
Congenital hip dislocation, 73, 170, 299
Constipation, 88, 122, 132-133
Contraception
  after childbirth, 303
  conceiving after stopping, 12-14
  and future pregnancy, 4, 12, 13
  see also specific contraception
Contractions
  Braxton Hicks, 158, 198, 209, 240
  see also Labor

Internal examination, 115, 208-209
Intrauterine device, *see* IUD
Intrauterine growth retardation
    (IUGR), 123, 155, 161
Intrauterine transfusion, 121
Iron supplements, 31, 40, 116, 127
Irwin, June, 52
IUD, 5, 12, 15-16

Jaundice
    in newborn, 121, 288, 296
    in pregnancy, 136
Jogging, 51, 53, 55, 197, 240
Junk food, 128

Kaopectate, 132
Kerenyi, Dr. Thomas, 216
Kidney disorder, 116
Kinship, and marriage, 79-80, 163-
    164

Labia, 87, 139
Labor, 247-252
    and anesthesia, 261-267
    back, 249, 250
    diagnosing onset of, 216-218, 243-
        244
    and electronic fetal monitors for
        distress, 253
    frequency of contractions in, 217
    and the hospital, 244-246
    "incoordinated," 263
    induced, 224-226
    and intercourse, 241-242
    and maternal distress, 252
    monitoring fetal distress during,
        253-259
    monitoring fetal heart rate during,
        253, 254-257
    natural, 219
    pain, 219
    pain-relieving drugs for, 259-261
    precipitate, 250
    premature labor, *see* Premature
        labor

prolonged, 250
    and rupture of membranes, 217-
        218
    walking during, 248
Lactation, 125, 295
Lactation, 125, 295
La Leche League, 294-295
Laminaria, 19
Lanugo, 207
Lasers, working with, 58
Lawrence, Andrea Mead, 52
Lead, exposure to, 61
Leboyer delivery, 159
Leg swelling, 287
"Let-down" response, 296
Leukemia, 4
Libido, 86, 144, 155, 300
Librium, 140-141
Lifting, 61, 65-66
Limb defects, 130
Linea nigra, 86
Lithium, 141
Local anesthesia, 134, 267
Lochia, 285-286
Low birth weight, 33, 34-35, 36-37,
    60, 123, 129
LSD, 38-39
Lungs, of immature infant, 223-224
Luteo-placental shift, 100, 154

Maalox, 133, 138
Malaria vaccine, 151
Marathon running, 53
March of Dimes, 80, 83, 167-168
Marijuana, 4, 7, 36-37
Masturbation, 147
Maternal distress, 252
Maternal mortality, 252
Maternity leave, 239
Mauriceau-Smellie-Veit maneuver,
    270
Meat, uncooked, 63
Megavitamins, 128
Meiosis, 69